The Nuts and
Bolts of
ICD Therapy

The Nuts and Bolts of ICD Therapy

Tom Kenny

Vice President Clinical Education & Training
St Jude Medical, Austin, Texas

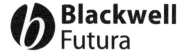

Published by Blackwell Publishing
Blackwell Futura is an imprint of Blackwell Publishing
Blackwell Publishing, Inc., 350 Main Street, Malden, Massachusetts 02148-5020, USA
Blackwell Publishing Ltd, 9600 Garsington Road, Oxford OX4 2DQ, UK
Blackwell Science Asia Pty Ltd, 550 Swanston Street, Carlton, Victoria 3053, Australia

First published 2006

Library of Congress Cataloging-in-Publication Data

Kenny, Tom, 1954-
The nuts and bolts of ICD therapy / Tom Kenny.

   p.;cm.
Companion v. to: The nuts and bolts of cardiac pacing.
Includes bibliographical references and index.
ISBN 978-1-4051-3511-5 (pbk.: alk. paper)

1. Implantable cardioverter-defibrillators. 2. Arrhythmia-- Treatment.
[DNLM: I. Defibrillators, Implantable. 2. Arrhythmia--therapy. WG 330 K36n 2006] I.
Kenny, Tom, 1954- Nuts and bolts of cardiac pacing. II. Title.
RC684.E4K46 2006
617.4'120645--dc22

                                                  2005026821

A catalogue record for this title is available from the British Library

Acquisitions: Gina Almond
Development: Simone Dudziak
Set in 9.5/12 pt Minion by Sparks, Oxford – www.sparks.co.uk

For further information on Blackwell Publishing, visit our website:
cardiology web: www.blackwellcardiology.com

Notice: The indications and dosages of all drugs and devices in this book have been recommended
in the medical literature and conform to the practices of the general
community. The medications described do not necessarily have specific approval by the Food
and Drug Administration for use in the diseases and dosages for which they are recommended.
The package insert for each drug. or device, should be consulted for use and dosage as
approved by the FDA. Because standards for usage change, it is advisable to keep abreast of revised
recommendations, particularly those concerning new drugs and devices.

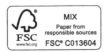

Contents

Preface, vii

1 Sudden cardiac death, 1

2 The history of ICDs, 12

3 The ICD system, 16

4 Indications for ICD implantation, 20

5 Implant procedures, 26

6 Sensing, 37

7 Arrhythmia detection, 43

8 Arrhythmia therapy, 50

9 SVT discrimination, 62

10 Bradycardia pacing, 70

11 Electrograms, 77

12 Special features, 86

13 Diagnostics, 93

14 A systematic guide to ICD follow-up, 106

15 Troubleshooting, 115

Glossary, 123

Index, 137

Preface

When I first started my clinical career, implantable defibrillators were 'dream machines.' We could understand in theory how they might work, but the technological obstacles seemed insurmountable. Now, halfway through my career, these devices are not only possible, they are almost commonplace. The technical restrictions that once seemed overwhelming are gone. Today's ICDs (implantable cardioverter defibrillators) are smaller than some of the pacemakers I once worked with! Despite the fact that a modern ICD is only about one-tenth the size of the original devices pioneered in the 1980s, these new devices last longer and do more.

In the early years of ICD therapy, it was practically a miracle that anyone ever qualified for an ICD. Indications required patients to have survived sudden cardiac death or SCD – not once, but twice! On top of that, patients had to be refractory to drug treatment and yet strong enough to survive an open-chest implantation procedure. Nevertheless, increasing numbers of patients received ICDs.

Today, we know that ICDs are not just a treatment of last resort for people with multiple documented episodes of ventricular fibrillation. As ICDs proved their mortality benefits to patients with known potentially lethal arrhythmias, investigators looked at other arrhythmia-rich populations. As a run of large randomized clinical trials has proven, ICDs have been shown to reduce mortality in primary prevention patients, that is, patients with no documented arrhythmias. Expanding ICD indications have saved lives by extending the proven mortality benefits of devices to more and more people. But this has simultaneously caused an interesting problem for the healthcare community: how can we care for this new influx of patients?

That's why this book was written. More and more clinicians are going to be confronted with managing ICD patients or at least understanding the role of the ICD in their care. Yet medical schools rarely devote much time to the subject of device-based therapy. Most so-called 'device experts' got their status through on-the-job training and the help of colleagues who taught them bits and pieces along the way. There are many fine books on device-based therapy for the heart, but many are written for the experts, not the newcomer.

With expanding ICD indications and hundreds of thousands of potential new ICD patients in the coming years, there are bound to be a lot of 'newcomers' to the care of the ICD patient!

Whether you're a rookie in terms of ICD therapy or whether you're just an occasional player, this book is a good place to start. Whether you read it cover-to-cover or use it for reference (or both), it was written primarily with you in mind. In my own experience, I learned about defibrillation from on-the-job mentoring from knowledgeable colleagues. Mentors are invaluable, and I'm glad to say it's a bit of a tradition in clinical practice. You may also find support and training opportunities through device manufacturers. I wrote this book to be one part of the solution for helping the busy clinician manage ICD patients.

Even if you're a veteran of ICD therapy, it is my hope that you'll find this book contains tips, pointers, facts, and information to which you'll want to refer. I have worked in various capacities in the field of device-based therapy since before there even were ICDs … and I am still learning about defibrillation. This book is not an in-depth volume for device experts; it's the nuts and bolts of ICD therapy for people who actually are involved in the clinical care of these patients.

No book is ever the work of one person. I have to thank my editorial team of Jo Ann LeQuang and Alan Yurkevicius for helping me put this manuscript together and my publisher, Blackwell, for ongoing support and encouragement. But most of all I want to thank my family for their continuing understanding for a busy husband and father who just had to take on one more project. For my wife Diane and our children, Christine, Brian, David, Matthew and Kevin, I want to express my love and affection for such generosity.

Tom Kenny
July 20, 2005
Austin, Texas

CHAPTER 1

Sudden cardiac death

Sudden cardiac death (SCD) – also known as sudden cardiac arrest (SCA) – has been defined as the unexpected natural death from a cardiac cause within a short time period from the onset of symptoms in a person without any prior condition that would appear fatal.[1] SCD has been described as an 'electrical accident of the heart,' in that SCD is a complex condition which requires the patient to have certain pre-existing conditions and then certain triggering events in order to occur. SCD is responsible for about 400 000 deaths a year in the US.[2] Despite our growing knowledge about the mechanisms and markers of this killer disease, SCD remains difficult to treat because the first symptom of SCD is often death.

Many risk factors have been identified for SCD. About 80% of those who suffer SCD have coronary artery disease (CAD), and the incidence of SCD parallels the incidence of CAD (men have CAD and SCD more often than women do, for example). One distinction is that while both CAD and cardiac-related death increase with age, *sudden* cardiac death decreases with age versus *nonsudden* cardiac death (NSCD). Older individuals are more likely to experience NSCD than SCD. The peaks of incidence of SCD occur in infants (birth to 6 months) and again between ages 45 and 75 years.[1]

Several risk factors have been identified for SCD. Some of them are the usual risk factors for any form of heart disease: smoking, inactivity, obesity, advancing age, hypertension, elevated serum cholesterol, and glucose intolerance. Anatomical abnormalities have been associated with SCD. For instance, acute changes in coronary plaque morphology (thrombus or plaque disruption) occur in the majority of cases of SCD cases; about half of all SCD victims have myocardial scars or active coronary lesions.[3] For people with advanced heart failure, a nonsustained ventricular arrhythmia was found in one study to be an independent predictor of SCD.[4] One report bolstered the popular belief that emotional distress can bring on SCD, in that it was found that the incidence of SCD spiked in Los Angeles right after the Northridge earthquake in 1994.[5] Other risk factors include the presence of complex ventricular arrhythmias, a previous myocardial infarction (MI) (particularly post-MI patients with ventricular arrhythmias) and compromised left ventricular systolic function. A low left ventricular ejection fraction is a risk factor that affects people with and without CAD. SCD survivors with a left ventricular ejection fraction < 30% have a 30% risk of dying of SCD in the next 3 years, even if they are not inducible in an electrophysiology study. If these patients are inducible to a ventricular arrhythmia despite drugs or empirical amiodarone, the risk can climb to as high as 50%![6]

SCD typically involves a malignant arrhythmia. In order for SCD to occur, a triggering event must occur which then has to be sustained by the substrate long enough to provoke the lethal rhythm disorder. The vast majority of SCD cases occur in people with anatomical abnormalities of the myocardium, the coronary arteries, or the cardiac nerves. Typical substrates are anatomical (scars from previous MIs, for example) but electrophysiologists also recognize *functional* substrates (such as those created by hypokalemia or certain drugs). By far the most common structural abnormalities are caused by CAD and its aftermath, the heart attack or MI. Cardiomyopathy is estimated to be the substrate for about 10% of SCD cases in adults.[7] Many people possess the substrates or conditions that make an SCD possible, yet they will never experience the disease. This is because SCD requires a triggering event which not only must occur, it must be sustained on the substrate long enough to develop into a deadly arrhythmia.

Reentry is by far the most common electrophysiologic mechanism involved in SCD. Reentry occurs when a natural electrical impulse from the heart gets 'trapped' in a circular electrical pathway in such a way that the impulse keeps re-entering the circuit, faster and faster, provoking a disordered and rapidly accelerating cardiac arrhythmia.

If the human heart were electrically homogenous, reentry and SCD could not occur. The healthy heart has electrical heterogeneity, which means that at any given moment, some cardiac cells are conducting while others are resting. At any point in time, different areas of the healthy heart are at different stages in the electrical cycle. To understand this better, it is useful to review the basics of cellular depolarization, repolarization, and membrane potential.

Action potential

All cells in the human body are covered with a semipermeable membrane that selectively allows some materials to penetrate into the cell while filtering out others. For cardiac cells, the membrane allows charged particles (ions) to flow in and out of the cell at specific times. By regulating the inflow and outflow of ions (electrical charge), cardiac cells are capable of generating and conducting electricity.

Even at rest, a cell in the heart has a certain number of ions within it that give it what scientists would call an 'electrical potential.' Electrophysiologists refer to this measurable electrical charge as 'membrane potential,' in that it is the electrical potential contained within the cardiac cell's membrane. The action potential describes five phases (numbered 0 through 4) that show how a cardiac cell goes from resting membrane potential (about –90 millivolts or thousandths of a volt) through depolarization, repolarization, and back to resting membrane potential (see Fig. 1.1).

In its resting state (phase 0), a cardiac cell contains a large quantity of negative ions (anions). Positive ions (cations) outside the cell are blocked from entering by the cell's membrane but they line up around the cardiac cell, attracted to the negatively charged particles within. It almost appears as if the inside of the heart cell was a negative pole and the immediate exterior of the cardiac cell was the positive pole. From this situation where opposites attract, the term 'polarization' is given. The charges

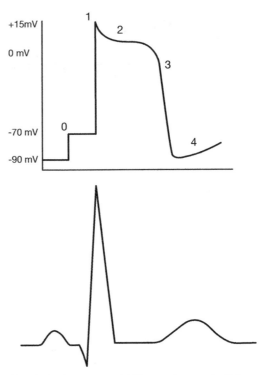

Fig. 1.1 Membrane potential. The membrane potential of a cardiac cycle involves five distinct phases (0 through 4) with phase 1 corresponding roughly to the peak of the R-wave.

polarize negative against positive. The membrane potential phases go from this polarized state (resting membrane potential) to depolarization, then repolarization, and back to the polarized state (resting membrane potential) (see Fig. 1.2).

When an electrical impulse reaches a cardiac cell, the cardiac cell membrane becomes permeable to positively charged sodium ions. Attracted by the negative pole within the cell, sodium ions rush into the cell until the interior of the cell is less negative and the exterior immediately around the cell's membrane is less positive. This shift decreases the cell's resting membrane potential to the point where fast sodium channels open in the cell membrane. Fast sodium channels are just like they sound; they allow a very rapid influx of positively charged sodium ions into the cell. As a result, the interior of the cell becomes positive and the exterior around the cell becomes negative. This phase – where polarization is reversed – is called depolarization.

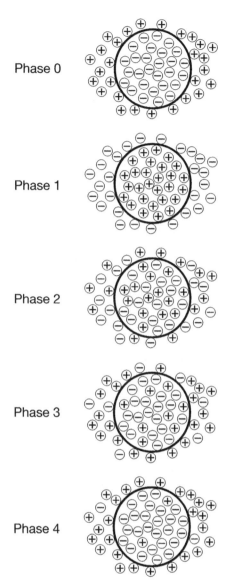

Fig. 1.2 Polarization of a cardiac cell. In phase 0 of the action potential, the cardiac cell contains a majority of negative ions within the cell with positive ions clustered around the immediate exterior. As ion channels open, positively charged ions rush into the cell (changing the cell's polarization or 'depolarizing' it). Positive ions flow back out using sodium as well as potassium and calcium channels, 'repolarizing' the cell to its original status.

The main physiological effect of cardiac depolarization is that the heart cells contract. That's why electrophysiologists frequently refer to the squeezing or pumping action of the heart muscle as 'depolarization,' since that best describes what is going

on in the heart's cells. At the cellular level, cardiac cells are becoming positively charged on the interior, negatively charged on the exterior – and this results in a heart beat.

The very process of contraction begins the next phase of the membrane potential, in that the positively charged sodium ions start to leave the inside of the cardiac cell when the cell contracts. Electrophysiologists call this process of getting back to the original resting membrane potential 'repolarization,' and it is characterized physiologically by the heart returning to a relaxed or resting state. At the cellular level, the positive ions flow out while negative ions flow back in using sodium as well as calcium and potassium channels. It is impossible for the cardiac cell to depolarize again until it has completed all three phases involved in repolarization; during phases 1–3, the cardiac cell is refractory.

The final phase of the action potential (phase 4) might best be viewed as a brief moment of rest. At the cellular level, there is very little activity going on, with only a few ions crossing the cell membrane either way (see Fig. 1.3).

The morphology of the action potential varies depending on the type of cardiac cell involved. Phase 0 shows how quickly the cell depolarizes, while phases

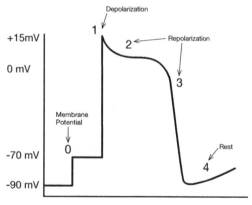

Fig. 1.3 Action potential. The action potential is an electrical way of describing the cellular changes that occur during depolarization and repolarization. At phase 0, the cardiac cell has a certain potential electrical energy. This ramps up quickly during phase 1 or depolarization when the cell rapidly changes polarity. Repolarization occurs more gradually in phase 2 and 3. There is a brief vulnerable period in phase 4 as the heart rests before resuming its membrane potential (phase 0) and starting the cycle over again.

1–3 show how long the refractory period is. The action potential from some main locations in the heart show that cardiac cells are specialized in terms of how fast they depolarize and how long they remain refractory (not able to depolarize) (see Fig. 1.4).

Automaticity

Automaticity is the heart's ability to spontaneously generate electricity. The specialized cells in the

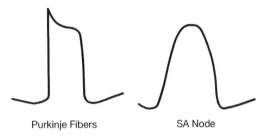

Purkinje Fibers   SA Node

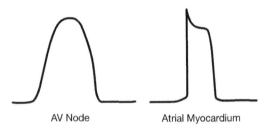

AV Node   Atrial Myocardium

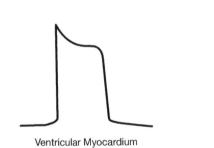

Ventricular Myocardium

Fig. 1.4 Action potentials of various portions of the heart. The action potential varies with the electrical activity of specific types of cardiac cells. Note that an atrial myocardial action potential is much narrower (briefer in duration) than a ventricular myocardial action potential. The rounded curves of the AV and SA nodal action potentials suggest that the transition from depolarization (phase 1) to repolarization (phases 2 and 3) is not as marked and abrupt as the same change in the Purkinje fibers. These illustrations show the different electrical properties of various regions of the cardiac tissue, which cause them to conduct electricity differently.

heart's sinoatrial (SA) node possess this remarkable property. The SA node is sometimes called the heart's 'natural pacemaker' for its ability to keep the healthy heart beating properly. Other myocardial cells possess automaticity and may spontaneously deliver an electrical output. In fact, many regions of the heart, including the atrioventricular (AV) node and even ventricular tissue, possess enough automaticity to 'fire' an electrical output. However, the heart's conduction system requires the electrical output to travel a specific path through the heart. At any given moment, the electrical pathway can only accommodate one output, and the heart works on a first-come, first-served principle. (In the cardiac conduction system, the fastest impulse wins.) The first output that gets on track is the one that travels. Other cells might generate an electrical output based on the principle of automaticity, but the pathway they will travel is refractory (not subject to depolarization because it is in phase 1, 2, or 3 of the action potential) and thus, the electricity will have no effect on the cells.

Automaticity and triggered automaticity are two of the three main causes of tachycardia, although altogether they account for only about 10% of all tachycardias. Automaticity involves abnormal acceleration of phase 4 of the action potential, causing the heart to launch into another depolarization too quickly. Its cause is increased activity across the heart's membrane in phase 4, usually involving a mechanism known as the sodium–potassium pump. As such, automaticity and triggered automaticity tachycardias have metabolic or cellular causes, and since they are not caused electrically, they do not respond to defibrillation. In fact, tachycardias caused by automaticity cannot be reproduced in the electrophysiology lab. The main causes of automatic tachycardias are thought to be ischemia (diseased heart tissue caused by CAD), electrolyte imbalances, acid/base imbalances, drug toxicity, and myopathy (muscle disorder).

It is often possible to observe the locations and types of cardiac disturbances by viewing variations in the action potential. Triggered automaticity looks a lot like reentry tachycardia on the action potential. It occurs when something triggers an automaticity-type tachycardia. A typical trigger might be a bradycardic pause or a catecholamine imbalance. This trigger accelerates phase 4 of the action potential,

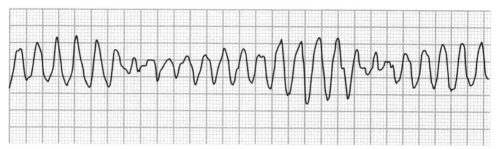

Fig. 1.5 Torsades-de-pointes. This is one of the best known types of ventricular tachyarrhythmia caused by triggered automaticity. Its name means 'twisting points', taken from the apparent twisting motion of the waveforms on an ECG. Torsades-de-pointes occurs when a trigger falls in the vulnerable phase 4 of the action potential, causing the heart to start its next depolarization too quickly (and thus accelerating the heart rate).

causing the heart to launch the next depolarization too quickly, resulting in an accelerating heart rate. A common example of triggered automaticity is the *torsades-de-pointes* type of tachycardia. Torsades-de-pointes (twisting points) takes its name from the French and describes the twisting or turning action the ECG seems to show (see Fig. 1.5).

Reentry

By far the most common mechanism for tachycardias anywhere in the heart is reentry, responsible for about 90% of all tachycardias. Although common, reentry is a complex mechanism which requires several specific conditions to be met before it can occur.

Reentry tachycardia first requires a bypass tract. The conduction pathway through the heart (from SA node over the atria to the AV node then out across the ventricles) is ideally a series of relatively straightforward unidirectional pathways from origin to termination. An impulse entering the pathway travels down through the cells, creating a cascade effect of depolarization and repolarization. Electrical impulses that enter the pathway after the initial impulse may still travel, but they encounter only refractory cells and cause no depolarization. A bypass tract occurs when the conduction pathway forms a branch that splits but then reconnects. As a result impulses traveling down the pathway may go down one side or the other, but will eventually regroup at the end (see Fig. 1.6).

For reentry to occur, this bypass tract must have a fast path and a slow path, that is, the two arms of the bypass tract must be electrically heterogeneous, that

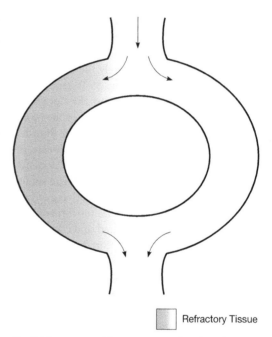

Refractory Tissue

Fig. 1.6 Bypass tract. A bypass tract consists of an electrical conduction pathway which splits at one point and then reconnects. This bypass tract allows electrical energy to flow down either the right side or left side of the tract. If both sides of the tract conducted electricity at exactly the same speed, this would not be a problem. However, if one side conducts electricity faster than the other side, it means that the cardiac tissue on one side of the bypass tract is going to be refractory at the same time as the other side is capable of conducting electricity. This means that electrical energy can get 'trapped' in the loop and circulate around and around the tract rather than flowing downward and out.

is, they must conduct electricity at different speeds. This, in turn, means that the two pathways will have different refractory periods. Impulses will travel more quickly through one path than the other, and one pathway can be refractory (not subject to depolarization) at the same time as the other pathway is depolarizing.

Finally, a reentry tachycardia requires some sort of triggering event, most commonly a premature contraction. This trigger enters the bypass tract and sets off a chain of events, which results in an endless loop of accelerating depolarizations, causing a very rapid heart rate (see Fig. 1.7).

Types of tachycardia

Supraventricular tachycardias (SVTs)

Supraventricular tachycardias (SVTs) originate above the ventricles and allow impulses to travel downward via the His-Purkinje network. SVTs can be caused by either automaticity or reentry mechanisms, and they are rarely life-threatening. When caused by automaticity, SVTs tend to be chaotic and multifocal, meaning they originate from many points in the upper areas of the heart. Usually caused by some sort of metabolic disorder (including digitalis toxicity, pulmonary disease, or acute alcohol poisoning), automatic SVT does not respond to pacing or cardioversion but can sometimes be reversed by treating the underlying cause.

Reentrant SVT is the more common form of SVT and may be congenital or acquired, and is known to occur even in patients without heart disease or acute illness. Intra-atrial reentry tachycardias (atrial flutter, atrial fibrillation) are caused when the reentry circuit occurs within the atria. SA or AV nodal reentrant tachycardias are sometimes also described as micro-reentry tachycardias because the whole bypass tract resides entirely in the SA or AV node – a very small ('micro') area.

AV nodal reentrant tachycardia (AVNRT)

AV nodal reentrant tachycardia (AVNRT) accounts for about 60% of all atrial, narrow-complex tachycardia seen in clinical practice, excluding atrial fibrillation. This micro-reentry tachycardia does not actually involve the atria or ventricles directly, since the whole bypass tract is contained in the AV node. On the other hand, the micro-reentry circuit in the

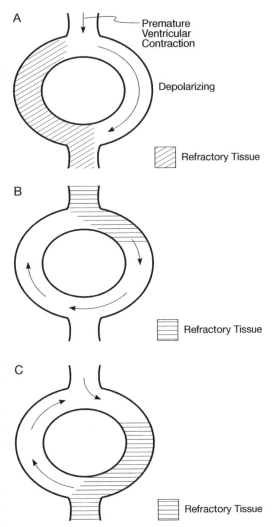

Fig. 1.7 Reentry tachycardia. Here is how a reentry tachycardia can get started. (A) A premature contraction or trigger enters the bypass tract. Since it is not properly timed (it arrives too early), it finds that tissue on one leg of the path is refractory. (B) The conduction on the fast path arrives at a juncture where it can either go down or back up. If it were not for the premature contraction, it would only be able to go down because the slow path of the bypass tract would all be refractory. However, the premature contraction has caused only part of the slow path to be refractory (shaded). This means that the electrical impulses in the fast path may travel back up and around the tract. (C) Because it is a loop, the bypass tract allows one impulse to keep traveling around and around the circuit. It accelerates as it does and causes rapid contractions of cells. New impulses can enter, but since the principle of cardiac conduction is 'fastest impulse wins,' the new impulses cannot take control.

AV node activates atria and ventricles, so the heart's upper and lower chambers both participate. One characteristic of AVNRT is that premature beats in one chamber do not affect the timing of beats in the other chamber.

Wolff-Parkinson-White (WPW) syndrome

In contrast to a micro-reentry circuit, sometimes a reentry tachycardia relies on a very large 'macro'-reentry circuit. An example of this is Wolff-Parkinson-White (WPW) syndrome where the bypass tract is large enough to connect the atrium directly to the ventricle. In this sort of tachycardia, the premature beats of one chamber will obviously advance the activation of the other chamber, since the bypass tract links atrium to ventricle.

Atrial fibrillation (AF)

The most common arrhythmia in the world is a type of intra-atrial SVT known as atrial fibrillation (AF). At one time, AF was described as chaotic atrial activity from multiple focal points, but modern theory holds that AF may actually be a more organized rhythm disorder than originally suspected. Many AF rhythm disorders originate in or near the pulmonary veins and not directly in the atria. AF is often inducible in the electrophysiology lab, but even there it can be hard to terminate. There are three broad classifications of AF, but even experts sometimes disagree as to where one category ends and the next begins. The three types of AF are paroxysmal (which terminates on its own), persistent (which requires medication, cardioversion, or both to terminate) and permanent (which cannot be stopped). While AF is not necessarily a lethal rhythm disorder in the same way that ventricular fibrillation is deadly, AF is associated with a greatly increased risk of stroke and other major health risks.

SVTs with rapid ventricular response

Patients with different types of SVT are typically treated with drugs to prevent the onset of the rhythm disorder or to slow down the ventricular response. Some SVTs can be treated with ablation, in which the reentry circuit is surgically destroyed. Ablation can be done by radiofrequency (RF), such as AV nodal ablation or by open-chest surgery (the Maze procedure). Newer, minimally invasive, catheter-based ablation procedures are being introduced.

Ablation still poses considerable clinical challenges in terms of mapping (finding the bypass tract) and navigation (getting to it), but when properly done in the appropriate patient, ablation is curative.

SVTs can also be treated with external cardioversion and defibrillation. Implantable atrial cardioverter-defibrillators are plausible devices that were in development in the 1990s, but they failed to gain widespread acceptance.[8] For the most part, SVTs are not lethal and some are even asymptomatic. An implantable device that dispenses an uncomfortable therapy to treat these SVTs was perceived as painful and intrusive by most patients.

Monomorphic and polymorphic VT

Ventricular tachycardia (VT) describes any too-fast heart rhythm that originates in the ventricles. Generally defined as occurring at rates between 100 and 300 beats a minute, VT can be monomorphic (originating from one focus in the ventricle) or polymorphic (originating from multiple focal points in the ventricle).

Monomorphic and polymorphic VT are fairly easy to detect on a surface ECG. Monomorphic VT consists of rapid but fairly regularly shaped QRS complexes. In monomorphic VT, all of the complexes should look similar in terms of complex morphology. On the other hand, polymorphic VT is characterized by differently shaped QRS complexes (see Figs 1.8 and 1.9).

VT can also be described as sustained (over 30 seconds in duration) and nonsustained (less than 30 seconds in duration). Nonsustained VT (NSVT) is a short run of VT which spontaneously terminates and is usually asymptomatic. Sustained VT lasts for a longer period of time, but may also spontaneously terminate.

Ventricular fibrillation (VF)

By far, the most lethal arrhythmia in the world is ventricular fibrillation (VF), which usually occurs at rates between 200 and 300 beats a minute. Unlike VT, in which clearly discernible (if somewhat erratically shaped) QRS complexes can be seen, VF is a wildly disorganized rhythm with no clear, individual QRS complexes at all. When VF occurs, the heart is no longer really pumping; it's quivering. Cardiac output drops to zero and the patient quickly approaches hemodynamic collapse. VF causes

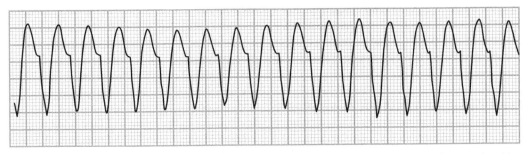

Fig. 1.8 Monomorphic VT. In a monomorphic VT, the tachyarrhythmia originates from a single place in the ventricles. This results in a series of QRS complexes which look similar to each other.

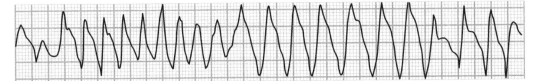

Fig. 1.9 Polymorphic VT. In a polymorphic VT, the tachyarrhythmia originates from more than one region in the ventricle. This causes the QRS complexes on the QRS to have different shapes, depending on their points of origin.

asystole (flat line) and leads to death, sometimes in as few as 4 minutes from time of onset. Fortunately, VF can be effectively reversed with timely defibrillation (see Fig. 1.10).

About 10% of all cases of VT have automaticity as the mechanism. An automatic VT is evidenced by an abnormal acceleration of phase 4 of the membrane potential. Ischemia and metabolic causes (electrolyte imbalance, acid/base imbalance) are the main causes of automatic VT, which can also be induced by drug toxicity. If the underlying cause of the automaticity can be addressed, automatic VT is completely reversible.

Long QT syndrome (LQTS)

Probably the best example of a VT involving triggered automaticity as a mechanism is long QT syndrome (LQTS). Although relatively rare, LQTS has received some attention in the cardiology community, particularly for an inherited form of the disease

which strikes families and often causes premature deaths of children and adolescents. While there is a divergence of opinion on the appropriate role of ICDs (implantable cardioverter-defibrillators) in this population, there is evidence that ICD implantation even in young people with congenital LQTS is appropriate.[9] While high-risk patients with congenital LQTS may benefit from ICD therapy, its use is controversial and some investigators advocate concomitant beta-blocker therapy.[10]

LQTS may also be acquired. On the membrane potential curve, LQTS affects the repolarization phase of the slope of phases 1–3. This prolongs the refractory period and allows a window of opportunity for intruding abnormal rhythms.

Torsades-de-pointes

Torsades-de-pointes is an example of a triggered-automaticity polymorphic VT and is often treated with magnesium infusion (even if serum magne-

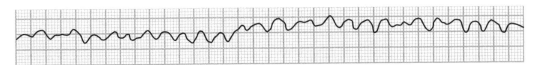

Fig. 1.10 Ventricular fibrillation. The most lethal of all arrhythmias, ventricular fibrillation lacks discernible QRS complexes. The tracing typically shows small-amplitude, bizarrely shaped signals that indicate a disorganized, quivering type of rhythm.

sium levels are normal), isoproterenol infusion or electrical rhythm management. Torsades-de-pointes is not a reentry tachycardia and is typically treated with pharmacological therapy. This type of arrhythmia is much more common in females than males, but the pathogenesis of torsades-de-pointes is not completely understood.[11]

Brugada syndrome

Brugada syndrome was first described just 10 years ago and has been the subject of considerable interest and study. A hereditary disorder, Brugada syndrome affects the early repolarization phase of the action potential (phases 1–2) and triggers a VT or even VF by automaticity. The disease exists all over the world, but is particularly prevalent in Asia. While more research needs to be done to better understand why a genetic mutation causes triggered automaticity in the ventricles, Brugada syndrome may respond to ICD therapy (see Fig. 1.11).[12]

Reentry VT/VF

By far the most common mechanism for VT and VF is reentry.[13] Reentrant VT frequently starts around an area of scar tissue on the heart, such as might occur as a result of an MI or heart disease. This scar area forms what cardiologists sometimes call the 'substrate' or area of compromised tissue that can support a reentrant VT or VF.

For patients who have had an MI, it is easy to understand how substrates form. During an MI, the heart muscle is deprived of valuable oxygen-rich blood. This lack of oxygen results in the necrosis or death of certain areas of cardiac tissue. The damage caused by an MI depends on where this tissue necrosis occurs and how much tissue is involved. Heart attack survivors have portions of diseased or scar tissue in the heart muscle. It is around this scar tissue that the conduction defect can occur. The dead tissue no longer conducts, but the margin of viable tissue around the scar often acts as aberrant conduction pathways. This is such a prevalent method for reentry tachycardia that all heart attack survivors should be counseled about their potential susceptibility to rhythm disorders.

In theory, reentry VT and VF can be treated by ablation, that is, the surgical removal of part of the bypass tract. The practical realities of VT ablation are much different: the bypass tracts are difficult to

locate and map and often involve a large area. Even if the bypass tract could be properly identified and surgically excised, the ablation procedure creates a new scar … and this can restart the cycle!

Medications to affect the action potential and slow the rate of conduction (thus reducing the heart rate and stopping or at least making the VT less severe) or drugs that change the refractory period (to inhibit reentry) have long been a mainstay in cardiology. However, most cardiologists know that cardiac drugs are toxic at incorrect dosages, require careful monitoring even at correct dosages, and sometimes have pro-arrhythmic effects. Implantable defibrillators, first introduced in the 1980s and pioneered in the next decade, offer real promise in treating VT and VF. The idea behind defibrillation

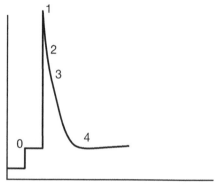

Brugada Syndrome

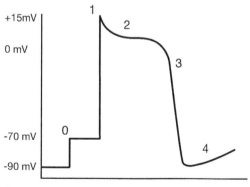

Fig. 1.11 Action potential for Brugada syndrome. The action potential for Brugada syndrome shows a very steep, almost immediate voltage decline after depolarization when contrasted to a normal action potential. Reentrant tachycardia occurs because of this shortened action potential.

is to treat the electrical cause of reentry VT/VF with a generic 'dose' of electricity. The implantable device was pioneered to make sure it was constantly on standby, ready to administer electrical energy whenever a potentially dangerous reentry ventricular arrhythmia occurred.

References

1 Zipes DP, Wellens HJJ. Sudden cardiac death. *Circulation* 1998; **98**: 2334–51.

2 State-specific mortality from sudden cardiac death – US 1999. From http://www.cdc.gov/mmwr/preview/mmwrhtml/mm5106a3.htm (downloaded March 14, 2005).

3 Theroux P, Fuster V. Acute coronary syndromes: unstable angina and non-Q-wave myocardial infraction. *Circulation* 1998; **97**: 1195–206.

4 Doval HC, Nul DR, Grancelli HO *et al.* Nonsustained ventricular tachycardia in severe heart failure: independent marker of increased mortality due to sudden death. *Circulation* 1996; **94**: 3198–203.

5 Leor J, Poole WK, Kloner RA. Sudden cardiac death triggered by an earthquake. *N Engl J Med* 1996; **334**: 413–19.

6 Weinberg BA, Miles WM, Klein LS *et al.* Five-year follow-up of 589 patients treated with amiodarone. *Am Heart J* 1993; **125**: 109–20.

7 Tamburro P, Wilber D. Sudden death in idiopathic dilated cardiomyopathy. *Am Heart J* 1992; **124**: 1035–45.

8 Ayers GM, Griffin JC. The future role of defibrillators in the management of atrial fibrillation. *Curr Opin Cardiol* 1997; **12**: 12–17.

9 Goel AK, Berger S, Pelech A, Dhala A. Implantable cardioverter defibrillator therapy in children with long QT syndrome. *Pediatr Cardiol* 2004; **25**: 370–8.

10 Monnig G, Kobe J, Loher A *et al.* Implantable cardioverter-defibrillator therapy in patients with congenital long-QT syndrome: a long-term follow-up. *Heart Rhythm* 2005; **2**: 497–504.

11 Surawicz B. Torsades de pointes: unanswered questions. *J Nippon Med Sch* 2002; **69**: 218–23.

12 Nemec J, Shen WK. Congenital long QT syndromes and Brugada syndrome: the arrhythmogenic ion channel disorders. *Expert Opin Pharmacother* 2001; **2**: 773–97.

13 Antzelevitch C. Basic mechanisms of reentrant arrhythmias. *Curr Opin Cardiol* 2001; **16**: 1–7.

14 Cupples LA, Gagnon DR, Kannel WB. Long- and short-term risk of sudden coronary death. *Circulation* 1992; **85** (Suppl I): 11–18.

The nuts and bolts of sudden cardiac death

- Sudden cardiac death (SCD), also known as sudden cardiac arrest (SCA), is one of the leading killers of Americans and remains a difficult disease to treat, because its first symptom is often death.
- There are many known risk factors for SCD including – but not limited to – coronary artery disease, smoking, inactivity, obesity, increasing age, hypertension, high cholesterol, and glucose intolerance.[14]
- Many malignant arrhythmias require a substrate or alternate conduction pathway in the heart and a triggering event to initiate a dangerous rhythm disorder.
- Reentry tachycardias occur when an electrical impulse gets 'trapped' in a bypass tract (substrate) and goes faster and faster, causing the heart to try to beat more and more rapidly.
- Automatic tachycardias are not caused by an electrical problem but occur when the heart tries to depolarize too quickly after repolarization,
usually as a result of an acid/base imbalance, electrolytic imbalance, metabolic condition, or some form of drug or alcohol poisoning.
- The action potential describes what happens in the heart at the cellular level that causes it to beat. The action potential consists of five phases (0 through 4) in which 0 involves depolarization, phases 1, 2, and 3 describe repolarization and the short phase 4 describes a brief moment of rest. Many cardiac conditions and the mechanisms of action for many cardiac drugs involve changes to one or more phases of the heart's action potential.
- Membrane potential is the electrical potential of a cardiac cell at rest.
- Automaticity refers to the ability of many types of cardiac cells to spontaneously generate electricity. Although the sinoatrial (SA) node is the heart's 'natural pacemaker,' many cells, including some in the AV node and others in the ventricle possess automaticity as well.

Continued.

Continued.

- Torsades-de-pointes is a form of automatic tachycardia and does not respond to electrical therapy.
- Most arrhythmias are named for where they originate (a supraventricular tachycardia is any too-fast rhythm that originates above the ventricles; it may affect atria and ventricles).
- For reentry to occur, there must be a bypass tract with a fast path and a slow path. This means that one portion of the tract will be refractory (that is, unable to depolarize) at the same moment that the other pathway is depolarizing.
- AV nodal reentrant tachycardia is a form of micro-reentry tachycardia because the reentry circuit is very small and entirely contained in the AV node. Wolff-Parkinson-White syndrome (WPW) is a form of macro-reentry tachycardia in that the reentry circuit directly links atrium to ventricle and covers a very large area of the heart.
- Two of the most common atrial arrhythmias are AV nodal reentrant tachycardia and atrial fibrillation.
- Atrial fibrillation (AF) is roughly classified into paroxysmal (sudden onset, terminates spontaneously), persistent (longer episodes that require intervention, typically drugs or cardioversion, to terminate) and permanent (refractory to treatment). AF is a progressive disorder.
- In general ventricular tachycardia (VT) is a too-fast heart rhythm that originates in the ventricles with a rate between 100 and 300 beats a minute. Ventricular fibrillation (VF), which is far more dangerous, is a too-fast, wildly disorganized heart rhythm that originates in the ventricles with a rate between 200 and 300 beats a minute or even higher. In terms purely of rate, it can be difficult to say if a ventricular tachyarrhythmia of 250 beats a minute is VT or VF without looking at an ECG. On an ECG, VF is a chaotic, disorganized rhythm and it is impossible to see a clearly differentiated QRS complex. VT, on the other hand, can be very fast but does show discernible QRS complexes.
- A monomorphic VT is one that originates from one source in the ventricle and all QRS complexes have a similar shape on the ECG. A polymorphic VT originates from more than one source in the ventricle and has different QRS morphologies present on the ECG.
- Long QT syndrome (LQTS) is a relatively rare disorder in which triggered automaticity causes ventricular fibrillation. It can be acquired or hereditary.
- Brugada syndrome is a hereditary disorder which provokes an automatic VT or even VF. It is more common in people from Asia and South America, and it may respond to defibrillation.

CHAPTER 2

The history of ICDs

Although the implantable cardioverter-defibrillator (ICD) is now an integral therapy for cardiac patient care and has saved hundreds of thousands of patients worldwide, its history is full of strife. As the first alternative to drugs and surgery, the ICD has faced formidable opposition and even today is not widely understood and endorsed by many clinicians outside of cardiology and electrophysiology.

Its inventor, Mieczyslaw (Michel) Mirowski was born in Poland in 1924. At age 14 he was forced to flee his home to escape the Nazis and was the only member of his family to survive the holocaust.

After the war, he attended medical school in Lyon, France. He completed his residency in Israel, and cardiology fellowships at the Johns Hopkins Hospital in Baltimore and the Institute of Cardiology in Mexico City. He returned to Israel in 1962 to become the Chief of Cardiology at Asaf Horofeh Hospital.[1]

In 1966 a friend and colleague of Mirowski, Professor Harry Heller, was diagnosed with recurrent ventricular tachycardia (VT). His sudden death, only 2 weeks later, inspired Mirowski's idea of implanting an automatic defibrillator. Although the concept for an automatic implantable defibrillator (AID) was born in Israel, the technology and funding necessary to develop it were not available there.[2] The first device implanted in a human was called an automatic implantable defibrillator or AID. However, it was later felt that this acronym implied that ventricular fibrillation (VF) was the only arrhythmia that the device treated, so the name was later modified to AICD (automatic implantable cardioverter-defibrillator) and subsequently shortened in popular usage to ICD.

In 1968 Mirowski became Director of the Coronary Care Unit at Baltimore's Sinai Hospital and in 1969 he began his research on the ICD with Dr Morton Mower. Though Mirowski was completely convinced that internal catheter defibrillation would work, his idea was rejected by almost everyone, including his own research partner Mower! In 1979 they published their first manuscript on the ICD and the medical community's response was one of severe denunciation. The sharpest criticism came from Dr Bernand Lown, the leading authority on defibrillation. He wrote in an editorial published in *Circulation* in 1972 that it was not only impossible to develop an ICD but unethical to test its performance since this required having to induce potentially lethal VF in the patient receiving such a device.[3] Lown did not foresee that ICD therapy would one day progress to the point where devices could be implanted under conscious sedation without the need for defibrillation threshold testing.

Mirowski garnered some initial support from a leading pacemaker company, but in 1972 this cooperation was terminated because of *a perceived lack of interest of the medical community in such a device*. Undaunted, Mirowski persisted and eventually met Dr Stephen Heilman who owned a small biomedical engineering company. After 2 years of work with this company, Mirowski and Mower developed the first implantable prototype and began testing in the animal lab, specifically with dogs. The system performed well in the canine tests, and could even recycle and deliver a second shock if the initial shock failed. In 1975 Mirowski and Mower made a film in which the implanted device resuscitated a dog from an induced VF.[4]

It wasn't until the mid-1970s that a series of 25 long-term chronic canine implants demonstrated the viability of the device. Films made of conscious animal testing showed that the device could sense and defibrillate VT effectively. In more than 60 implants, there were only four failures, all attributable to lead damage associated with surgical technique.

Clearly, ICD therapy showed promise, yet the investigators still received no support from the scientific community, who doubted the data's veracity and even challenged the dog movies as fakes! Subsequent films of animal tests ran simultaneous ECGs, but even this did not convince the critics.

Only after extensive investigational review board inquiries did the team get permission for human implants. Even then, patients had to meet almost impossible entry criteria: a patient had to have survived at least two life-threatening ventricular arrhythmias (which were not within 6 weeks of documented myocardial infarction – MI) plus they must have failed pharmacological therapy.[3]

The first ICD patient was a 57-year-old woman with documented coronary artery disease, a history of acute MI, and recurrent syncope with documented VF. She had failed extensive drug testing and she and her family agreed to try device therapy. She underwent general anesthesia on February 4, 1980 at Johns Hopkins Hospital with Dr Levi Watkins as the operating surgeon. The procedure was going quite well, until the ICD was requested. The circulating nurse picked up the package containing the device and dropped it to the floor! The device was damaged and could not be implanted in the patient. Fortunately, a second device was available, and it was successfully implanted without complications.

The report of the first human implant was published in *The New England Journal of Medicine*.[5] From 1980 to 1985 the device then known as the AID was implanted in some 800 patients at institutions on both sides of the Atlantic, including the Fundación Jiménez Díaz in Spain.

Finally, in 1985, 19 years after Michel Mirowski first conceived the idea for the device, the FDA cleared the ICD for commercial sale in the US.[6]

Tribute and recognition followed. In 1989 the Mirowski Symposium was begun as a way to honor the pioneering work of Dr Michel Mirowski in the development of the implantable cardioverter-defibrillator and to further the understanding of the emerging field of electrophysiology. Traditionally the Mirowski Award is given during this program to recognize an individual who has made vital contributions to the understanding of cardiac rhythm disturbances.[6] In 1990 Mirowski died, but his legacy to the world, the ICD, literally lives on in the hundreds of thousands of patients whose lives are prolonged by them. In 2002 Michel Mirowski was inducted into the National Inventors Hall of Fame for his pat-

ent number 4,202,340 Method and Apparatus for Monitoring Heart Activity, Detecting Abnormalities, and Cardioverting a Malfunctioning Heart.[7]

Over 20 years have passed since the first ICD implant. ICD therapy has significantly decreased sudden cardiac death (SCD) from arrhythmia (VT and VF).[8] Primary treatment trials have shown ICD therapy to be superior to drug therapy for many patient populations. Ongoing trials include evaluation of ICD therapy for patients in such arrhythmia-rich populations as patients with congestive heart failure,[9] dilated cardiomyopathy,[10] hypertrophic cardiomyopathy,[11] and repolarization syndromes.[12] Factors such as medication inefficacy/side effects and overwhelming mortality benefits have expanded ICD usage beyond the original restrictive guidelines.[13] (See Fig. 2.1.)

The first ICDs required a thoracotomy to implant. The original defibrillation leads were epicardial patches, large mesh conductors that were sutured to the outside of the heart (see Fig. 2.2). While epicardial patch leads were safe and effective, the highly invasive implantation procedure conferred some risk to patients considering ICD implant. Often, ICDs were only implanted in patients undergoing other open-chest procedures. In addition, devices were very large and could only be comfortably implanted in the abdomen. A tunneling tool was required to route the epicardial lead down to the generator, where it plugged in. An ICD implant procedure could take several hours and required considerable expertise on the part of the physician. The invention of the transvenous defibrillation lead along with the radical downsizing of the generator allowed the ICD to be implanted in a minimally invasive procedure with the generator placed pectorally and leads routed transvenously, in the same manner as pacemaker leads. This invention made ICD implantation faster, safer, and technically easier, and it opened up the benefits of ICD therapy to a wider base of potential patients.

Despite bitter criticism, much opposition and even bad luck, the ICD has succeeded in becoming a major life-saving component of modern cardiac medicine. The need to educate clinicians about ICD and its benefits remains one of the greatest challenges in getting ICDs to all of those who need and can benefit from them. The cardiac community should find inspiration in Dr Mirowsky's tenacity as we

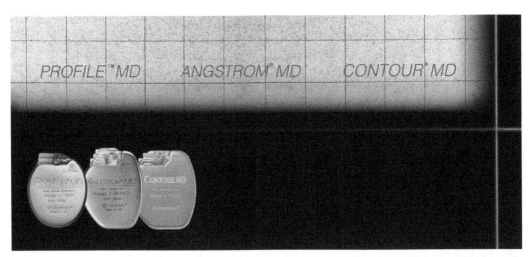

Fig. 2.1 Downsizing ICDs. Although the largest device in this series, the Contour® ICD, was considered to be 'downsized' when it was released in the early 1990s. ICDs have continued to get smaller and smaller until today, they approach the size of older-generation pacemakers. Courtesy of St Jude Medical.

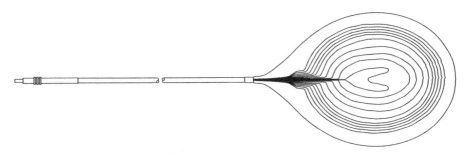

Fig. 2.2 Epicardial patch lead. The earliest leads were 'patch' leads which were designed to be sewn onto the exterior of the heart in a thoracotomy.

persevere in increasing our own knowledge as well as sharing it with other clinicians and patients.

References

1 http://www.invent.org/hall_of_fame/175.html (accessed April 28, 2005).

2 http://www.mamweb.org/modules.php?name=Content&pa=showpage&pid=44024 (accessed April 28, 2005).

3 Lown B, Axelrod P. Implanted standby defibrillators. *Circulation* 1972; **46**: 637–9.

4 http://www.mamweb.org/modules.php?name=Content&pa=showpage&pid=44024 (accessed April 28, 2005).

5 Mirowski M, Reid PR, Mower MM *et al.* Termination of malignant ventricular arrhythmias with an implanted automatic defibrillator in human beings. *N Engl J Med* 1980; **303**: 322–4.

6 http://www.mamweb.org/modules.php?name=Content&pa=showpage&pid=44024 (accessed April 28, 2005).

7 http://www.guidant.com/mirowski/ (accessed April 28, 2005).

8 Shah AH, Huang DT, Rosero SZ, Daubert JP. Update on implantable cardioverter-defibrillator trials. *Curr Cardiol Rep* 2004; **6**: 327–32.

9 Bardy GH, Lee KL, Mark DB *et al.* Sudden cardiac death in heart failure (SCD-HeFT) Investigators. Amiodarone or an implantable cardioverter-defibrillator for congestive heart failure. *N Engl J Med* 2005; **352**: 225–37.

10 Grimm W, Alter P, Maisch B. Arrhythmia risk stratification with regard to prophylactic implantable defibrillator therapy in patients with dilated cardiomyopathy. Results of MACAS, DEFINITE, and SCD-HeFT. *Herz* 2004; **29**: 348–52.

11 Kuck KH. Arrhythmias in hypertrophic cardiomyopathy. *Pacing Clin Electrophysiol* 1997; **20**: 2706–13.

12 Perkiomaki JS, Couderc JP, Daubert JP, Zareba W.

Temporal complexity of repolarization and mortality in patients with implantable cardioverter defibrillators. *Pacing Clin Electrophysiol* 2003; **26**: 1931–6.

13 http://www.heartdiseasej.com/pt/re/heartdis/ abstract.00132580-200205000-00007.htm;jsessionid= CeeMDu2nmQ5LhYtarOFVEsjbjZ1ubXjviSOrMSeJZ NOtdEkiKM1Q!2000813083!-949856031!9001!-1 (accessed April 28 2005).

The nuts and bolts of ICD history

- The ICD has not always enjoyed acceptance as a medical treatment of first resort, but clinical evidence has gradually expanded indications for its use.
- Dr Michel Mirowski is generally credited as the inventor of the ICD, inspired to create a life-saving device by the sudden cardiac death of a dear friend.
- The idea for the ICD was 'born' in Israel, but developed in the US.
- The first devices were called AIDs or automatic implantable defibrillators. This name was changed when it was feared some might think it treated only ventricular fibrillation and not ventricular tachyarrhythmias. A new name – implantable cardioverter-defibrillators – was coined, the abbreviation of which is used today (ICD).
- Mirowski's early canine experiments with defibrillation (captured on film) were at one time denounced as a hoax by some individuals in the medical community.
- The first human implant of an ICD occurred in 1980. By 1985, about 800 devices had been implanted in the US and Europe.
- The FDA gave market clearance to the first ICD in 1985. These early devices required a thoracotomy to place epicardial leads and the large generator had to be placed abdominally.
- Innovations to the ICD, particularly transvenous defibrillation leads and a radically downsized generator, have encouraged greater use of the ICD.
- Dr Mirowski died in 1990 but the Mirowski Symposium and Mirowski Award honor his memory.

CHAPTER 3

The ICD system

The initial concept of an implantable device capable of providing therapy to a fibrillating heart dates back to 1966, when pacemakers were relatively new, yet rapidly gaining clinical and patient acceptance. Some of the technology from pacemakers migrated readily to the implantable cardioverter-defibrillator (ICD). For example, ICDs consisted of electronic components and a battery housed in a hermetically sealed titanium case. A clear epoxy header on the top of the device connected to the internal battery and 'brains' of the system through metal feedthroughs. The leads plugged into the header, were secured with a set-screw or other mechanism, and then allowed device energy to travel through the feedthroughs into the leads and on to the heart.

The electronic components of the pacemaker are created on a hybrid circuit, a small board which contains a variety of transistors, resistors, chips, and other components connected to provide proper electrical timing. As devices got more advanced, the components were more similar to a miniature computer. They could not only provide electrical stimulation according to predefined algorithms, they could modify their responses based on the patient's own heart beats. Even more advanced devices would incorporate a memory function so that sensed information could be stored in the device and downloaded later through a proprietary table-top computer known as a programmer.

Like a pacemaker, the implantable defibrillator had to be a self-contained, battery-powered device. Specially designed lithium-vanadium cells had emerged as an ideal ICD battery. (These are cousins of the lithium-iodine batteries used in pacemakers.) Lithium is a very light metal with what engineers call the highest standard potential, meaning that lithium has the highest energy density. Lithium cells are not widely used for household or industrial purposes because lithium reacts violently when exposed to water and can only be used when the battery is hermetically sealed.

In battery technology, lithium (the metal) serves as the anode or positive pole and another element acts as the cathode or negative pole. For pacemakers, iodine (a trace mineral) was found to be a suitable cathode. (Lithium and iodine are the substances, but when they react together they are lithium-iodide.) Lithium-iodide cells were small, lightweight, and had very predictable, reliable discharge curves, that is, they produced energy in a predictable way.

Some of the early ICDs used the lithium-iodide battery technology of their pacemaker cousins, but a new lithium-vanadium battery soon emerged as the preferred battery for ICD devices. (There are many other types of lithium batteries as well.) Vanadium is a trace element which acts as the cathode in these cells. Like lithium-iodide batteries, lithium-vanadium cells are powerful, long-lived batteries with reliable discharge curves.

One of the most significant technical hurdles to overcome in creating an implantable defibrillator was finding a suitably large battery. Pacemakers typically pace at outputs of 1–3 volts, sometimes even less than that. Since the lithium-iodide cells in use were around 2.4 volts, these batteries worked well. Components called voltage multipliers could take the voltage produced, ramp it up, and allow the device to deliver as much as a 7 (or in some devices, even 10) volt output. Such high outputs were rare and most pacemakers use a voltage multiplier to increase voltage only slightly.

The defibrillating energy delivered by an ICD was hundreds of times that amount. In fact, ICDs can deliver 500, 700 or more volts in a single therapy delivery. While it was possible to use larger batteries to get more voltage, the initial technological barrier was finding a battery that was small enough yet could deliver hundreds of volts to a patient – all on a few seconds' notice!

The problem was solved with an electronic component called a capacitor. Unlike voltage multipliers, which could only augment a small amount of voltage, a capacitor was designed to hold a charge and deliver it all at once. One way to think of a capacitor is as a bucket, which the battery keeps filling with voltage until sufficient voltage is in the bucket. At that moment, the bucket is tipped over and all of the voltage is delivered at one instant.

Early capacitor technology still required a relatively large battery, plus the device had to be large enough to accommodate the capacitor – not a miniature component. As devices progressed, capacitors got smaller, smarter, and then flatter. Today's ICDs are no bigger than the pacemakers of the 1970s. However, the original units were quite large and might weight 700 or 800 grams (a modern ICD weighs about 70 grams).

The first ICDs only delivered defibrillation therapy. Later on, lower-voltage therapy known in the industry as cardioversion was added, which earned the devices their acronym: implantable cardioverter-defibrillator. Pacing support was a function not added to ICDs until the 1990s, but today almost all ICDs, including the most basic systems, offer pacing support. In fact, when ICDs are called 'single-chamber' or 'dual-chamber' systems, that distinction does not apply to the defibrillation capability of the unit; it refers to the type of pacemaker function the device provides. Single-chamber ICDs defibrillate the heart and offer VVI(R) pacing. Dual-chamber ICDs defibrillate the heart and offer DDD(R) pacing.

In order to deliver a high-voltage output to the heart, engineers were also challenged to design a special type of lead that would transmit the voltage from the device to the heart. The first generation of ICDs relied on epicardial leads, which were titanium-mesh 'fly swatter' leads made with Dacron® reinforced rubber. This mesh patch was sewn onto the outside of the heart in an open-chest procedure. In a typical procedure, two epicardial patches were sewn onto the heart: one in the anterior right ventricular region and the other in a posterior, lateral, left ventricular area. The idea was that current would flow through the mass of the heart from patch to patch.

While epicardial leads worked well, they required patients to undergo a thoracotomy in order to get an

ICD implanted. Once the patch leads were sutured to the heart, the proximal ends were 'tunneled' to the abdomen, where a pocket was created to hold the device. The tunnel was created with a tunneling tool that created a passageway for the leads to go from the heart via the abdomen to the device. Abdominal implants were common in the earliest ICDs, in fact, they were routinely performed through the mid-1990s. One reason an abdominal implant was the preferred method was the size and shape of the devices. They were very large, heavy, and rectangular and could not really be accommodated in other parts of the body.

Without a doubt, one of the greatest innovations in ICD technology was the development of a transvenous defibrillation lead. Unlike pacing leads, which were required only to pace and sense the heart (that is, deliver or receive small electrical signals), a defibrillation lead had to be able to deliver a large amount of electrical energy in a single output. The epicardial patches worked well for that purpose, but they made ICD implantation a major invasive procedure. A transvenous lead made the implantation much less invasive and greatly improved patient acceptance (see Fig. 3.1). It also helped move the process from one requiring general anesthesia to an

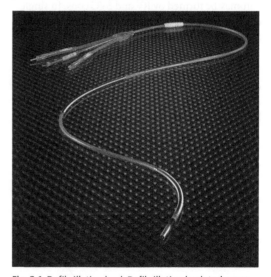

Fig. 3.1 Defibrillation lead. Defibrillation leads today are transvenous, meaning they can be implanted through the vasculature rather than requiring an open-chest procedure. Downsizing the lead diameter has led to the creation of reliable leads that can pace, sense, and defibrillate and which are comparable in size to bipolar pacing leads. Courtesy of St Jude Medical.

operation that could be done under conscious sedation and sometimes even on an outpatient basis.

In order to create a transvenous defibrillation lead, engineers had to create an electrical circuit capable of withstanding a large bolus of electricity. To do this, they created leads with a special 'coil' of wire capable of delivering a large jolt of electricity. Single-coil defibrillation leads use one coil, while dual-coil defibrillation leads had a proximal and a distal coil (much like the old epicardial system of using two points of energy). These leads were much thicker in diameter than conventional pacemaker leads, but they could still be passed through the vasculature and maneuvered into place in the right ventricle, where they were fixated (using either an active fixation or passive fixation mechanism) in the same manner as low-voltage pacemaker leads. Over time, technology allowed defibrillation leads to reduce their diameter until today, when they are not much larger than bipolar pacing leads (see Figs 3.1 and 3.2).

A defibrillation lead typically contains two coils, one at the distal end (the right ventricular or RV coil) and another, a bit more proximal than the far distal coil (the superior vena cava or SVC coil). Shocking energy travels along a circuit, and this circuit may be formed by RV and SVC coils. In single-coil leads, the circuit is formed from the RV coil to the device can.

In addition, today's defibrillation leads do more. Since most ICDs today also function as single-chamber or dual-chamber pacemakers, defibrillation leads today pace and sense like pacemaker leads but also come equipped with one or more coils to defibrillate the heart when necessary. Small-diameter defibrillation leads have made it easier than ever to implant a complete ICD system, even in smaller framed patients. Of course, in the rare cases when ICDs are required in pediatric patients, it may be necessary to use the epicardial patch leads since even the smallest available transvenous defibrillation leads could be too large for a small child.

ICDs are housed in a titanium case, sometimes nicknamed the 'can' (see Fig. 3.3). Titanium is a very light, extremely strong, biocompatible metal that had already established itself as a valuable material in pacemaker implants. An ICD 'can' is actually two halves. Components on a hybrid board, a battery, one or more capacitors, and other components are put in one half of the can; the other half is put on top to close the can and the two halves are laser-welded together in such a way as to create a hermetic seal. This seal protects the inside of the device from the invasion of bodily fluids.

One, two, or sometimes three leads plug into the clear epoxy header on top of the device. In the first generation of dual-chamber ICDs, it was common to implant a right atrial pacing lead, a right ventricular pacing lead, and a defibrillation lead in the right ventricle. Today, even dual-chamber ICDs rarely require

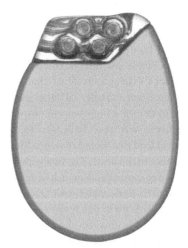

Fig. 3.3 Modern ICD. This ICD weighs only about one-tenth of what the first ICDs weighed and it offers far more functions and lasts longer. Advances in capacitor and battery technology have allowed for downsized, streamlined ICDs capable of full-featured dual-chamber pacing along with advanced defibrillation functions. Courtesy of St Jude Medical.

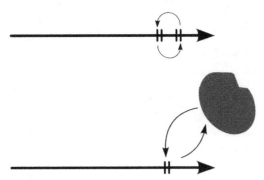

Fig. 3.2 Defibrillation leads. A single-coil defibrillation lead forms an electrical circuit from the coil on the lead itself to the ICD device (can). Dual-coil defibrillation leads form the electrical circuit from one coil to the other.

more than two leads, since the right ventricular lead both paces/senses and defibrillates the heart. In cases where there are more ports in the header than leads to be used, a silicone plug is provided to seal the opening of the device before it is implanted.

Devices communicate with clinicians through a proprietary table-top computer known as a programmer. A telemetry wand is placed over the implanted device and establishes bidirectional communication, allowing the device to download diagnostic data and other information (including stored electrograms) and allowing the clinician to change parameter settings. Long available for pacemakers, remote patient monitoring is now available for ICDs in the form of home-based transmitters that utilize wrist electrodes and either phone lines or Internet connections to send information. Such remote systems do not allow for a clinician to adjust the device, but can allow battery status and recent diagnostics, including recent therapy deliveries, to be checked.

Although ICDs are relatively new devices on the market, most of the anticipated innovation in this field involves advancements in the electronic components, memory storage capabilities, and capacitor technology. These innovations are creating devices that are more automatic, store more data for clinicians, or are smaller or longer-lived.

The nuts and bolts of the ICD system

- Today's ICD looks much like a pacemaker: a titanium-housed 'can' with a clear epoxy header with lead ports for lead connections. Like a pacemaker, it is a hermetically sealed device containing elaborate and sophisticated internal components.
- ICDs use lithium-vanadium batteries, similar to the lithium-iodine batteries used in pacemakers. These are reliable energy sources with predictable discharge curves.
- An ICD is able to deliver a charge larger than its battery voltage because it relies on a system of capacitors which hold a charge and then release it all at once when it is large enough.
- For an ICD, defibrillation is high-energy shock, while cardioversion is a low-energy shock.
- A single-chamber ICD offers single-chamber pacing capability, while a dual-chamber ICD offers dual-chamber pacing capability. The single-chamber and dual-chamber designations have nothing to do with the defibrillation capability.
- Early ICD leads were epicardial patch leads that required a thoracotomy in order that they could be sewn onto the exterior of the heart. Today's defibrillation leads are transvenous leads that are not much bigger in diameter than bipolar pacing leads.
- Shocking energy travels – like all energy flow – around a circuit (that is, in a circular path). If the defibrillation lead has two coils, then the circuit is formed from the far distal or right ventricular (RV) coil to the slightly more proximal coil or superior vena cava (SVC) coil. In single-coil defibrillation leads, the current pathway is from RV coil to the device can.
- Nothing simplified ICD implantation more than today's transvenous leads, downsized devices (suitable for pectoral implant) and more automated device programming. In fact, today ICD implantation can be done on an outpatient basis instead of requiring open-chest surgery!

CHAPTER 4

Indications for ICD implantation

The American College of Cardiology and the American Heart Association together with the Heart Rhythm Society (formerly known as the North American Society of Pacing and Electrophysiology) have issued official guidelines on ICD indications.[1] While these guidelines represent the consensus of medical opinion as to the use of ICDs, these guidelines are not legally binding on physicians. The Centers for Medicare and Medicaid Services (CMS) in the United States reach decisions on device coverage independently of these guidelines, which means that the consensus of medical opinion is not necessarily the same as what is covered by health insurance. The guidelines are best viewed in their proper context: they are guidelines reached by some of the leading experts in cardiac care. In actual practice, physicians must rely on their own clinical judgment as to what is best for an individual patient. Insurance coverage may not be available for certain otherwise recommended or advisable procedures. However, the guidelines are frequently cited and carry considerable weight in political, legal, and financial circles.

Guidelines use a class system for indications. A Class I indication is one for which the consensus of medical opinion holds that the treatment is beneficial and useful. A Class III indication is one for which general agreement holds the treatment is not useful, not effective, and might even be harmful. Class II is divided into Class IIa (conflicting evidence as to benefits with weight of evidence finding the treatment useful) and Class IIb (conflicting evidence as to benefits with weight of evidence finding the treatment not useful). See Table 4.1.

In the past decade, numerous randomized clinical trials have explored the use of ICDs in new patient populations. The first MADIT[2] trial and MADIT II[3] evaluated the use of ICDs in primary prevention patients, that is, patients who did not have a conventional ICD indication and, in fact, had never had documented sustained ventricular tachycardia (VT). The idea behind MADIT and MADIT II was to evaluate the potential benefits, if any, of prophylactic ICD implantation in patients who had not yet had an episode of sudden cardiac death (SCD). In the DEFINITE trial, ICDs were shown to reduce mortality in patients with nonischemic cardiomyopathy.[4] Both MADIT trials found that prophylactic ICDs significantly reduced the risk of all-cause mortality in these primary prevention patients. Subsequent trials, including SCD-HeFT,[5] found that ICDs reduced all-cause mortality in primary prevention patients

Table 4.1 Indications by class

Class	Defined as
I	Evidence and/or general agreement that ICDs are beneficial, useful and effective
IIa	Conditions for which there is conflicting evidence and/or a divergence of opinion about the usefulness or efficacy of a procedure or treatment, but where the weight of the evidence or opinion favors the usefulness and efficacy of the procedure or treatment
IIb	Conditions for which there is conflicting evidence and/or a divergence of opinion about the usefulness or efficacy of a procedure or treatment, but where the weight of the evidence or opinion does not find the procedure or treatment useful or effective
III	Conditions for which there is evidence and/or general agreement that a procedure or treatment is not useful or effective and, in some cases, might even be harmful

significantly compared with amiodarone (which did about as well as the placebo arm in this three-arm study). Numerous other studies have expanded our knowledge of who might benefit from ICD therapy. However, even a large randomized clinical trial with significant results does not necessarily result in an immediate change to official guidelines and it can take even longer before results from a clinical trial translate into coverage decisions.

Randomized clinical trials have improved our understanding of how devices work and what patient populations might benefit from ICD therapy, but it is important to view these results in context. Rarely is one study – even a very sound one – sufficient to change clinical opinion. Each new study seems to open up more questions. While it is now clear that ICDs do reduce mortality rates in arrhythmia-rich primary prevention populations such as heart attack survivors, new questions arise as to how to best quantify risk for individuals in the primary prevention groups. Another serious question in this regard involves the cost-effectiveness of ICD therapy. Even if we knew that ICD therapy reduced mortality rates in a certain population, is the healthcare system prepared to pay for ICDs in such patients? Medical literature contains several proposals as to how we might best define cost-effective ICD therapy, but there is no official opinion as to what constitutes cost-effectiveness in ICD therapy.[6–8]

Class I indications

These are considered indications for which ICD implantation is generally held to be a beneficial, useful and effective treatment.

- **Cardiac arrest due to VF or VT** not due to a transient or reversible cause. These patients are the so-called 'SCD survivors.' If the arrhythmia was caused by something temporary (for instance, being struck by lightning) or something that could be reversed (for example, an electrolyte imbalance), then this indication does not count. The thinking behind this indication is that any patient who suffered a potentially life-threatening ventricular arrhythmia remains at risk for the arrhythmia to return, unless there are specific reasons why it will not return.
- **Spontaneous sustained VT** in association with structural heart disease. The mere presence of VT is not an indication in and of itself. The VT must be sustained, that is, capable of lasting long enough to be dangerous to the patient, and the physician must understand the underlying physical mechanism that is supporting the ventricular arrhythmia. For many patients, this structural disease will be an arrhythmic substrate that could be identified in an electrophysiological (EP) study. Spontaneous VT differs from induced VT, in that spontaneous VT arises on its own without any external provocation.

- **Syncope of undetermined origin with clinically relevant, hemodynamically significant sustained VT or VF induced at EP study when drug therapy is ineffective, not tolerated or not preferred.** Patients with this indication must have had an EP study during which the electrophysiologist was able to induce not just VT or VF, but a ventricular arrhythmia that had hemodynamic and clinical consequences for the patient. If such patients experience episodes of syncope for unknown reasons, physicians can then make a clinical decision as to whether to treat this condition with drug therapy or a device. Note that for such patients, drugs are the first approach. An ICD is only indicated when the patient is inducible to significant VT/VF, has syncope of unknown origin, and drugs are not desired. While drugs are given first preference, an ICD may be selected if the physician or patient prefers device-based treatment to drug therapy. Many ICD patients are on appropriate, concomitant drug treatments.

- **Nonsustained VT in patients with coronary disease, prior MI, LV dysfunction, and inducible VF or sustained VT at EP study that is not suppressible by a Class I antiarrhythmic drug.** Nonsustained VT is a brief run of VT that terminates spontaneously (less than 30 seconds). Such episodes are not uncommon in a wide range of patients, particularly those with other forms of heart disease, and do not necessarily indicate the use of an ICD. This particular indication addresses patients with known heart disease (as evidenced by a prior heart attack, left ventricular systolic dysfunction and coronary artery disease) who also had drug-refractory sustained VT or VF in an EP study. The drug typically used in such studies is procainamide, although other Class I antiarrhythmics meet the guidelines.

- **Spontaneous sustained VT in patients without structural heart disease** not amenable to other treatments. This indication allows that patients with spontaneous runs of sustained VT might also benefit from ICD therapy if they are not amenable to other treatment options, notably drug therapy.

  These Class I indications encompass:
- SCD survivors;
- those with sustained VT (including those who have structural heart disease and those without structural heart disease who do not respond to other treatments);
- those inducible to sustained VT or VF in an EP study who have either;
  - unexplained syncope (and do not respond to or want to use drug therapy) or
  - episodes of nonsustained VT and coronary disease plus a prior heart attack and left ventricular dysfunction.

Class IIa

These are indications where there is some conflicting evidence or divergence of opinion, but where the weight of the opinion favors implantation of an ICD.

- **Patients with a left ventricular ejection fraction (LVEF) of less than or equal to 30% at least 1 month post-myocardial infarction (MI) and 3 months post-coronary artery revascularization surgery.**

  The LVEF is a commonly used index of systolic function. It basically refers to how much of the contents of the left ventricle is ejected or pumped out into the body during one cardiac cycle, stated as a percentage. As a rule of thumb, an LVEF of around 50% is normal. Many randomized clinical trials set an LVEF cut-off value of about 35% to describe left ventricular dysfunction. ICDs are indicated in patients with an LVEF of 30% or below providing they have had an MI and revascularization (usually at least 30 days previously). A person with a low LVEF score *but no prior heart attack* is not considered a Class IIa indication.

Class IIb

Class IIb indications include many categories of patients. For these groups, there is a divergence of opinion as to whether or not ICDs should be implanted, but the weight of the evidence argues that ICDs are not useful, effective or beneficial in these groups.

- **Cardiac arrest presumed to be due to VF when EP testing is precluded** by other medical conditions. Patients in this category survive sudden cardiac arrest (SCA) but are not fit to undergo EP testing which would conclusively prove that the SCA was caused by ventricular fibrillation (VF). It is possible that their SCA was caused by something other than VF.
- **Severe symptoms (e.g. syncope) attributable to ventricular tachyarrhythmias in patients awaiting cardiac transplantation.** This population describes a relatively small subset of patients who are on the list to receive a donor heart. In such patients, even extremely symptomatic VT is not an ICD indication.
- **Familial or inherited conditions with a high risk for life-threatening ventricular tachyarrhythmias such as long QT syndrome (LQTS) or hypertrophic cardiomyopathy.** We are just beginning to learn about some inherited diseases that put certain people at increased risk for ventricular arrhythmias, including LQTS, which typically appears in young people. As a Class IIb indication, the weight of the evidence holds that ICD implantation is not beneficial or effective in these groups.
- **Nonsustained VT with coronary artery disease, prior MI, left ventricular dysfunction, and inducible sustained VT or VF in an EP study.** Heart attack survivors with compromised left ventricular function who can be induced in an EP study to VT or VF are not considered to benefit from ICD implantation even if they experience runs of nonsustained VT.
- **Recurrent syncope of undetermined origin in the presence of ventricular dysfunction and inducible ventricular arrhythmias in an EP study when other causes of syncope have been excluded.** The weight of the evidence holds that patients who have compromised ventricular function, can be induced to VT or VF in an EP study and experience recurrent bouts of syncope (for which noncardiac causes have been ruled out) are considered not to benefit from ICD therapy.
- **Syncope of unexplained origin or family history of unexplained SCD in association with typical**

or atypical right bundle-branch block and ST-segment elevations (**Brugada syndrome**). We are just starting to learn about a condition known as Brugada syndrome. Although present all over the world, Brugada syndrome occurs most frequently in Asia and strikes young adults. Brugada syndrome is an inherited disorder that causes SCD, and is currently the subject of considerable clinical investigation. At present, the weight of medical evidence finds that ICDs are not effective in this particular population.

- **Syncope in patients with advanced structural heart disease in whom thorough invasive and noninvasive investigations have failed to define a cause.** One of the most confounding symptoms for clinicians is syncope, in that this potentially ominous symptom can trace back to a wide variety of causes, some benign. Investigating unexplained syncope can be difficult for clinicians, since this symptom may be impossible to recreate in the clinic or EP lab. The mere presence of syncope – even if no cause can be ascertained – is not an ICD indication (see below, Class III). But even patients with severe structural heart disease are not considered to benefit from ICD implantation if their syncope cannot be specifically traced to a cardiac cause.

Class III

The Class III indications include several patient populations for whom the consensus of medical opinion holds that ICD implantation is not beneficial or effective.

- **Syncope of undetermined cause in a patient without inducible ventricular tachyarrhythmias and without structural heart disease.** The mere presence of syncope for an unknown reason does not warrant ICD implantation if the patient is not inducible in an EP study and has no other evidence of some form of structural heart disease.
- **Incessant VT or VF.** A chronic ventricular arrhythmia is not an ICD indication. This form of tachyarrhythmia differs from spontaneous VT or VF which originates suddenly and can resolve spontaneously.
- **VF or VT resulting from arrhythmias amenable to surgical or catheter ablation,** for example, atrial arrhythmias associated with Wolff–Parkinson–

White (WPW) syndrome, right ventricular outflow tract VT, idiopathic left VT or fascicular VT. There are varieties of ventricular arrhythmias that respond better to ablation and for which medical opinion does not advocate the use of an ICD.

- **Ventricular tachyarrhythmias due to a transient or reversible disorder** (e.g. acute MI, electrolyte imbalance, drugs, or trauma) when correction of the disorder is considered feasible and likely to substantially reduce the risk of recurrent arrhythmia. Ventricular arrhythmias, even those causing severe symptoms, may occur due to a temporary condition such as hyperkalemia (potassium overload) or right after a heart attack. Patients with such arrhythmias are not indicated for ICD implantation if the condition can be reversed and that reversal will substantially reduce their risk of having the arrhythmia.
- **Significant psychiatric illnesses** that may be aggravated by device implantation or may preclude systematic follow-up. Even relatively stable patients may need some time to adjust psychologically to the presence of an implanted device that occasionally delivers high-energy shocks. Patients whose mental state would not allow them to cope with such a device or those who are unable to participate in their own therapy by appearing for regular follow-up appointments are considered inappropriate candidates for ICD treatment.
- **Terminal illnesses with projected life expectancy less than 6 months.** Many physicians caring for terminally ill patients who had earlier ICD implantations are now contending with the issue of when and under what conditions to disable the device. It is not appropriate to implant an ICD in a patient whose death is imminent.
- **Patients with coronary artery disease with left ventricular dysfunction and prolonged QRS duration in the absence of spontaneous or inducible sustained or nonsustained VT who are undergoing coronary bypass surgery.** Even patients with other related cardiac conditions, such as coronary artery disease, left ventricular dysfunction, and long QRS, are not considered candidates for ICD therapy if they cannot be induced to VT or VF in an EP study and have elected to submit to a coronary bypass graft.
- **NYHA Class IV drug-refractory congestive heart failure patients who are not candidates**

for cardiac transplantation. Class IV heart failure patients are the most severely symptomatic, in that their condition is defined as those patients with heart failure who experience heart failure symptoms (shortness of breath and fatigue) even at rest. While some heart failure patients are candidates for heart transplantation, many are not. But of these most severe heart failure patients, even the ones who are not otherwise eligible for a cardiac transplant, are not indicated for an ICD.

Indications review

ICD indications can be complicated because the indications are expanding in the wake of a variety of recent major scientific studies and because symptoms and conditions of the various classes are very similar.

For example, cardiac arrest is a Class I indication if the physician is certain the event was caused by VT or VF, but it becomes a Class IIb indication when an EP test cannot be conducted to prove that VT or VF was at the root of the problem. Syncope may be present in Class I, Class II, or Class III indications. The only time syncope is involved in a Class I indication is when the patient is inducible in an EP study to VT or VF and drug therapy is ineffective, not well tolerated or not preferred. For patients without structural heart disease who are not inducible in an EP study, syncope – even of unknown cause – is a Class III indication.

Conditions we are just beginning to understand, such as LQTS and Brugada syndrome are considered Class IIb indications, but in actual clinical practice, it is possible to encounter such patients who have received ICDs. Device implantation is always a matter of clinical judgment and the fact that a person may meet Class IIb rather than Class IIa conditions does not preclude the implantation of a device.

References

1   Gregoratos G, Abrams J, Epstein AE *et al.* ACC/AHA/NASPE 2002 Guideline update for implantation of cardiac pacemakers and antiarrhythmia devices: a report of the American College of Cardiology/AHA Association Task Force on Practice Guidelines, 2002. Available at acc.org (accessed June 18, 2005).

2   Moss AJ, Hall WJ, Cannom DS *et al.* Improved survival with an implanted defibrillator in patients with coronary disease at high risk for ventricular arrhythmia. Multicenter Automatic Defibrillator Implantation Trial Investigators. *N Engl J Med* 1996; **335**: 1933–40.

3   Moss AJ, Zareba W, Hall WJ *et al.* Prophylactic implantation of a defibrillator in patients with myocardial infarction and reduced ejection fraction. *N Engl J Med* 2002; **346**: 877–83.

4   Kadish A, Quigg R, Schaechter A *et al.* Defibrillators in nonischemic cardiomyopathy treatment evaluation. *Pacing Clin Electrophysiol* 2000; **23**: 338–43.

5   Bardy GH, Lee KL, Mark DB *et al.* Amiodarone or an implantable cardioverter-defibrillator for congestive heart failure. *N Engl J Med* 2005; **352**: 225–37.

6   O'Brien BJ. Chapter 3. Cost effectiveness of ICD therapy: a review of published evidence. *Can J Cardiol* 2000; **16**: 1307–12.

7   Hlatky MA, Sanders GD, Owens DK. Evidence-based medicine and policy: the case of the implantable cardioverter defibrillator. *Health Aff (Millwood)* 2005; **24**: 42–51.

8   Chen L, Hay JW. Cost-effectiveness of primary implanted cardioverter defibrillator for sudden death prevention in congestive heart failure. *Cardiovasc Drugs Ther* 2004; **18**: 161–70.

The nuts and bolts of ICD indications

- The decision as to who gets an ICD and who does not involves numerous constituencies, including government entities (regulatory bodies), health services (government entities), private insurance companies, physicians and their patients. The ACC/AHA/NASPE guidelines, last revised in 2000, are considered to represent leading medical opinion. However, these guidelines do not assure coverage for therapies and are not legally binding on physicians.
- The guidelines describe indications as Class I (consensus of medical opinion finds ICDs would be beneficial, useful, and effective) and Class III (consensus finds that ICDs would not be beneficial, useful, or effective). Class II involves a divergence of opinion with Class IIa favoring an ICD and Class IIb favoring no ICD.
- The existence of so many Class IIa and IIb device indications shows that, even among learned physicians, it is not entirely clear which patient populations will and will not benefit from ICD implantation.
- Randomized clinical trials have been expanding potential patient populations who have been clinically proven to benefit from ICD therapy. There can be a time lag between the conclusion of a large randomized clinical trial, its appearance in print, and the time taken for its findings to make their way to official guidelines. It usually takes even longer for such findings and guidelines to change coverage decisions. Since electrophysiologists enjoy the reputation of being 'early adopters,' it is often possible that physicians working with ICDs have already changed their clinical practice in response to new evidence before official coverage decisions are reached.
- Recent clinical trials have found that ICDs can reduce the risk of death in primary prevention populations.
- While incessant VT or VF is a Class III indication, spontaneous sustained VT in the presence of structural heart disease is a Class I indication.
- Cardiac arrest due to VT or VF is a Class I indication, but it is Class IIb if an EP study cannot be conducted to ascertain that VT or VF was indeed at the root.
- Ventricular arrhythmias, even if severe, are not indications for a device if they are caused by temporary conditions or things that might be corrected, such as drug use, acute myocardial infarction, or electrolyte imbalances.
- Syncope is a Class I indication only if the patient can be induced to significant VT or VF in an EP study and drugs are not the desired treatment modality. If the cause of syncope cannot be ascertained conclusively (either because it was not possible to do an EP study or because the EP study was negative), then it is a Class IIb indication if the patient also has structural heart disease. If that patient does not have structural heart disease, then it would be a Class III indication.
- Heart attack survivors with an LVEF less than or equal to 30% are now a Class IIa indication.
- Brugada syndrome and long QT syndrome are Class IIb indications.
- Patients expected to die imminently, those awaiting heart transplant, drug-refractory Class IV heart failure patients, and those with serious psychiatric disorders are not indicated for ICDs.
- The decision to implant a device is always a matter of clinical judgment on the part of the physician and many factors come into play. The guidelines are exactly that – guidelines rather than strict rules.

CHAPTER 5

Implant procedures

There is probably no better example of how technology has improved patient safety, reduced costs, and streamlined clinical procedures in cardiac rhythm management than in the area of ICD implantation. In 1985, the first ICDs were implanted using a thoracotomy (open-chest procedure) which required epicardial patch leads to be sewn onto the heart and the other end of the lead to be 'tunneled' to the device, which was so large it had to be placed in the abdomen. In 1993, transvenous defibrillation leads did away with the thoracotomy and allowed devices to be implanted in less invasive procedures. Today, the use of relatively small diameter defibrillation leads, radically downsized ICDs, and faster, more intuitive device testing has made it possible to implant an ICD almost as easily as a pacemaker. In 1985, an ICD implantation would take many hours and keep the patient hospitalized for a week or more. Today, ICD implantation is routinely done on an outpatient basis and when hospitalization is required it rarely involves more than an overnight stay.

Prior to implant

The very first stages of preparation for ICD implantation involve discussing the procedure and ICD therapy with the patient and family members. Despite the wealth of medical information available today, many patients will have misconceptions about device therapy or not have any idea what to expect.

The patient's medical history and diagnosis should be reviewed, along with results from any electrophysiologic (EP) studies. If the patient is taking some sort of anticoagulant, including aspirin therapy, this should be discontinued prior to the implant procedure to prevent complications from bleeding. Lab tests, including bleeding times, should

be assessed before the procedure to be sure that it is safe for the patient to undergo surgery. A routine chest X-ray, 12-lead ECG, and echocardiogram to assess left ventricular ejection fraction (LVEF) and valve status are also needed before surgery.

The physician should inspect the site that is being considered for implantation. In general, the left pectoral region is used, mainly because venous access is easier from this side. If the patient is left-handed or if there is some other reason for not using the left side, then the right pectoral region can be used.

Preparation for implant

In clinical practice, it is possible to observe ICD implantations in a wide variety of locations, including a fully equipped operating room (OR), a cardiac catheterization lab (CCL) or an electrophysiology lab (EPL). The hospital will determine where the procedure is to take place based on its own institutional guidelines and policies. More crucial than the place where the procedure takes place is the fact that the patient needs to be able to be moved into the Trendelenburg position in which the lower half of the body is elevated. In some cases, the physician may prefer to prop up the patient's legs with a wedge-shaped pillow. The Trendelenburg position is generally more comfortable for the patient and it encourages blood flow to the upper half of the body, plumping the cephalic and subclavian veins for easier venous access.

Emergency equipment (crash cart) should be available along with emergency medications. The room should be equipped with standard equipment, including an X-ray or fluoroscope, oxygen, suction, surgical instruments, and an appropriate sterile field.

For ICD implantation, the team will also need the ICD device and leads, plus back-up products (in the unusual event that there is something wrong with the first device). It is good policy to have at least one back-up for every sterile item, since unforeseen events can and do happen. A programmer with wand should also be available, with the wand placed in a sterile plastic pouch for use during the procedure. (It is not possible to sterilize the programmer, so putting the wand into a sterile bag and only allowing that portion of the system into the sterile field is the standard procedure.) A pacing system analyzer (PSA) should also be available along with the appropriate cables. Although they are not commonly used, it is good practice to bring along adapters, wrenches, plastic tools, or other small accessories.

The team

Implanting an ICD may be close to becoming 'routine surgery,' but it still takes a team of qualified and experienced clinicians to make it look easy. The implanting physician is typically an electrophysiologist or a surgeon. A nurse or anesthesiologist is included, who typically provides conscious sedation and a local anesthetic. In some cases, general anesthesia may be required. There is usually a scrub nurse and a circulating nurse available, as well as a representative from the manufacturer. In some facilities, there may be other clinicians as well, including a fluoroscopy technician.

The role of the manufacturer's representative in such procedures has long been familiar and appreciated by the clinical staff, but may be confusing or unexpected for the patient. Many facilities today require hospital officials to disclose the presence of the representative to the patient, who, in turn, may question this practice. The representative's role is to act as the official 'authority' on the device, leads, programmers and other equipment provided by their company. Representatives do not act as medical advisors, but may be needed to answer questions about device function and provide information (for example, if an adapter is required or if the patient's anatomy might preclude the use of a particular model of product). Device company representatives and the clinical staff work closely during all phases of care of ICD therapy, including implantation.

The representative may be asked to prepare the device for implantation. This involves a series of very easy but very important steps. First, the device should be interrogated while it is still in the box to confirm that it is off (that is, will not be able to deliver therapy and possibly shock the implanters) and that battery voltage is appropriate for a new device fresh out of the box. Devices with an expired 'use-before date' may not have the same amount of initial battery energy as a new device. (The 'use-before date' appears on the outer box of the ICD and represents the amount of shelf-life a device has before housekeeping current drain – that is, the amount of energy needed to maintain the device even when it is not activated – impacts the battery life. An expired 'use-before date' does not mean that the device is no longer sterile or will not work. It just does not have the full measure of battery life that a newer device would have, which may adversely impact device longevity. There are cases when it may be appropriate to implant such a device.)

The next step involves a simple capacitor maintenance charge. This allows the device to 'charge up' as if it were about to deliver therapy. During this test, the representative or technician should confirm the charge time, which should be within the specifications set forth by the manufacturer for a new device. Typically, this initial charge time should be 15 seconds or faster.

Using the programmer, the representative will program some initial parameters for the device to make it easier and quicker to implant. Bradycardia parameters (that is, pacing) should be enabled or programmed on, because real-time measurements will only be accessible when this is activated. DFT testing (described later) may be required after implantation and it may be expedient to program the type of DFT test desired at this point. If the representative does not know what the implanting physician might want or if the implanting physician changes their mind later on, the type of DFT test can be reprogrammed relatively easily. During this programming step, it is crucial that the tachycardia parameters of the device are not programmed on, since implanting a 'live' device exposes the physician and implanting team to a risk of shock.

Many ICDs allow for patient information to be programmed into the device itself using the programmer. If the representative has time at this point, the patient's name and any pertinent information (lead model numbers, date, and so on) can be entered into the device. During follow-up, the patient's name will automatically print out on programmer print-outs and other reports if it is entered into the device.

Venous access

Just like implanting a pacemaker, the first surgical step in the procedure involves identifying and accessing a vein for lead insertion. Successful ICD implanters use the internal or external jugular veins, the subclavian vein, the axillary vein, and the cephalic vein. The vein chosen by the implanting physician will depend largely on physician preference and the patient's anatomy. Most physicians use the cephalic or subclavian vein. When the cephalic vein is used, it is typical to use the 'cut-down approach,' that is, to identify, lift up, and then excise the vein. The subclavian vein can be accessed using the 'subclavian stick' in which a needle is used to puncture or 'stick' the subclavian vein. While both are commonly used and known to be safe and effective, there is probably a clinician preference, overall, for the cephalic cut-down technique (see Fig. 5.1).

A sheath or introducer is then inserted into the vein to allow for easy passage of the leads. The smallest possible diameter introducer should be used, since very wide diameter introducers may increase implant trauma, damage the vein, or cause back-bleeding or other complications.

The implanting physician will also create a pocket in the pectoral region large enough to accommodate the device snugly.

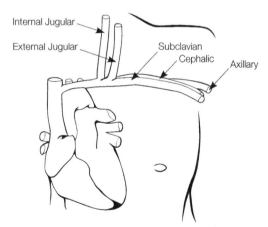

Fig. 5.1 Venous anatomy. Although it is possible to implant defibrillation leads using any number of veins, the cephalic and subclavian are the most commonly used vessels.

A defibrillation or tachycardia lead is inserted into the right ventricle. This is a very versatile lead in that it is capable of providing ventricular pacing, ventricular sensing, and high-energy defibrillation to the heart. This lead is inserted into the right ventricle and fixated in or near the ventricular apex.

A single-chamber ICD may require only one lead. Dual-chamber devices also require a lead to be placed in the right atrial appendage. This lead often has a preformed characteristic J-shape which aids in proper lead placement. Once properly located in the right atrial region, the lead is fixated to the atrium, often using an active fixation mechanism (corkscrew or helix mechanism).

Leads are guided through the introducer under fluoroscopic observation and fixated to the right ventricle or right atrial appendage. Once they are fixated inside the heart (using either passive fixation mechanisms such as tines or barbs or active fixation corkscrews) and get good values, the proximal end of the leads are plugged into the ports of the defibrillator. Depending on the type of device, the lead may be held in place by a set-screw or other mechanism designed to hold the lead firmly in the generator's clear epoxy header.

Lead testing

While the lead may appear to be placed appropriately, the implanting physician must check its performance in a series of tests. If the leads do not function as well as expected, moving or changing their position may be required. In many device procedures, it is not unusual to relocate the leads (even more than once) to find the best possible values. Using the small, hand-held pacing system analyzer or the programmer, the first test should involve assessing the P-wave and R-wave and checking lead impedance values. The R-wave, that is, the intrinsic ventricular signal, should be 5 mV or greater. The P-wave or intrinsic atrial signal should be 2 mV or greater (see Fig. 5.2).

Next, it is important to confirm that the pacing leads can capture or consistently and reliably depolarize the heart. A capture test should be performed for both chambers to obtain suitable values. Again, this corresponds to what is done during pacemaker implantation (see Fig. 5.3).

Real-time measurements should also be obtained to verify that all parameter settings are as anticipated.

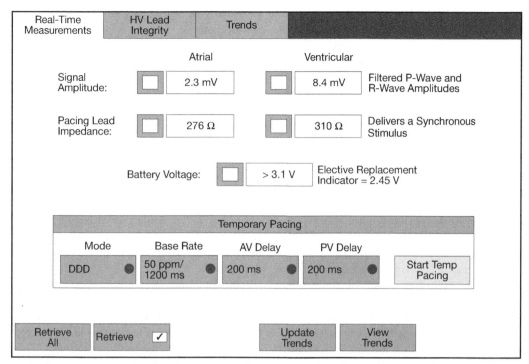

Fig. 5.2 Programmer screen at implant. In this example, the patient has a 2.3 mV atrial signal (P-wave) and an 8.4 mV ventricular signal (R-wave), both of which are large enough for good sensing characteristics in the device. Pacing lead impedance is 276 and 310 Ohms, respectively, which falls within range for this particular type of lead. This step of the procedure is similar to what goes on during a pacemaker implantation. Battery voltage is > 3.1 V, which is appropriate for a brand new device.

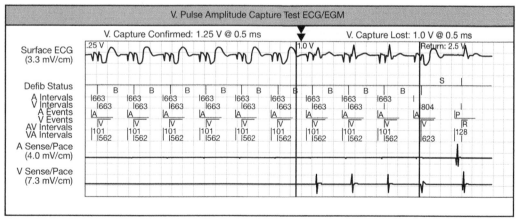

Fig. 5.3 Ventricular capture test. Capture thresholds should be tested for ICDs, just like for pacemakers. In this example, the patient's capture threshold was 1.25 V at 0.5 ms, which is an acceptable value.

Note that if the implanting physician feels that better values can be obtained by repositioning the leads, he or she will move the leads and re-test. This is not unusual in this sort of procedure and can contribute to better long-term device function.

Device-based testing (DBT)

Testing the pacing performance and pacing lead parameters of an ICD is relatively easy and straightforward. But it may also be important to test the defibrillation or shocking capability of the device, and this portion of the implant procedure is more challenging. Some ICDs allow for portions of the defibrillation testing to be automated, but this can be overridden so that a manually controlled test is conducted. Device-based testing (DBT) refers to the fact that the ICD itself contains features which allow it to self-test for defibrillation efficacy. During DBT, pacing output parameters (pulse amplitude and pulse width) are ramped up temporarily to maximum settings (7.5 V at 1.9 ms).

To conduct DBT, telemetry must be established using the programmer wand. If the wand is removed or telemetry is otherwise interrupted, the DBT procedure automatically terminates and the device reverts to previously programmed settings.

The first step in DBT is obtaining the impedance values for the defibrillation lead, sometimes called the high-voltage lead integrity check (HVLIC) (see Fig. 5.4). In this test, the ICD delivers a 12 J shock to the patient's heart through the defibrillation lead, synchronous to the heart's intrinsic activity. After the test, the programmer will report the lead impedance value, which should be appropriate for the particular system according to the manufacturer's specifications.

Although this self-test uses a relatively low 12 J shock, this is still something most patients find uncomfortable or even painful. For that reason, it may be important to warn the consciously sedated patient of an impending shock and to reassure them afterwards.

If impedance values are out of range, it indicates that there is a problem with the lead and its ability to deliver life-saving therapy. Impedance values that are too high suggest that the lead is not secured properly in the clear epoxy header or that the lead's conductor coil is broken or damaged. Impedance values that are too low suggest that the lead's outer insulation layer has been nicked or otherwise damaged.

If the impedance values are out of range and cannot be corrected (for example, by tightening the setscrews to hold the lead in place), the lead should be replaced. Further device testing should not proceed until high-voltage lead integrity is confirmed.

Before testing the device, it is important to program the tachycardia parameter settings. While these

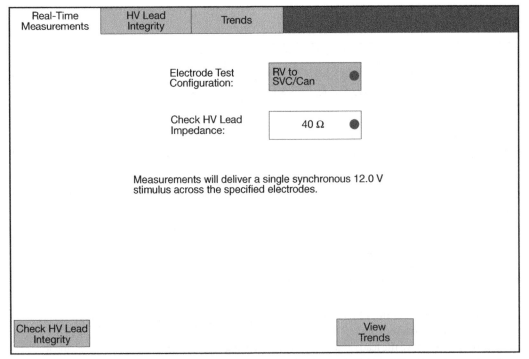

Fig. 5.4 High-voltage lead integrity check. The programmer reports that the result of this test is an impedance value of 40 Ohms, which falls well within range. Out of range impedance values suggest a problem with the lead.

are subject to review and revision, the basic parameter settings should be adjusted at this point. Most ICDs recommend certain nominal values which are effective in the majority of patients. These default settings are generally acceptable 'starting points' at this time.

Defibrillation threshold testing

The defibrillation threshold (DFT) is the minimum amount of energy required to reliably defibrillate the heart when it is experiencing a potentially life-threatening ventricular arrhythmia. Knowing the patient's DFT allows the physician and other clinicians to be sure that the ICD is programmed to deliver sufficiently high-energy shocks to defibrillate the heart.

In some cases, the implanting physician may opt to forego DFT testing because it is painful, time-consuming, and consumes battery energy. If the implanting physician intends to program the device to maximum output anyway, DFT testing (which would allow programming less than maximum output values) may not be worth the effort. Furthermore, many patients are likely to be shocked only rarely and then for serious situations. For such patients, programming maximum energy therapy is appropriate, and DFT testing is not necessary. Increasingly, DFT testing is omitted at implant. However, when performed, DFT testing can help physicians optimize the output settings of the device.

The goal of any DFT test is first to induce an arrhythmia and then to allow the device to shock the patient and convert the rhythm. If DFT testing is to be conducted, the anesthesiologist should be advised to administer deeper sedation, since this portion of the procedure is definitely considered painful. The entire team should be readied. At the programmer, it may be necessary to select options for DFT testing, since many devices offer a variety of ways to do this sort of testing.

Inducing the arrhythmia can be done through the device using a direct current shock (such as DC Fibber or other feature), a shock-on-T, or through burst stimulation. A direct current shock uses about 8 V of direct current delivered to the heart through the defibrillation lead. This is known to be a reliable way to induce fibrillation. Some physicians may prefer burst pacing, during which short-cycle bursts are delivered to the heart synchronously to the next sensed event or when the next pacing interval times out. This method is more similar to some EP induction methods relying on burst stimulation. The burst stimulation method delivers bursts through the pacing lead and is the only induction method available for atrial induction. (Although it is not common practice to induce atrial fibrillation during DFT testing, there may be occasions when atrial induction is required.) The shock-on-T mode overdrives the ventricle for 12 stimuli and then delivers a carefully timed high-energy shock.

The method of induction depends largely on physician preference as well as individual considerations for the particular patient.

Once fibrillation is induced, the device delivers high-energy therapy, and the patient is monitored to verify defibrillation. Since this is a testing phase, it is quite possible that defibrillation will not occur. For that reason, the implant team should be prepared before testing starts to deliver a rescue shock in the event of an unsuccessful therapy. If multiple shocks are required during DFT testing, the patient should be allowed to rest and recover for about 5 minutes between tests.

Most ICDs allow for semi-automatic DFT testing in that once fibrillation is induced, the device automatically relies on the programmed settings to detect the arrhythmia, diagnose it, and deliver therapy (see Fig. 5.5). After the shock is delivered, the intracardiac electrogram should be monitored to verify that:

- There was appropriate sensing during the episode.
- There was appropriate detection of the episode.
- The arrhythmia was converted.
- The delivered energy is known.
- Shocking impedance values are in range.
- Charge time (that is, amount of time between diagnosis and therapy) is acceptable; charge times should be at their quickest in a new device.

Of utmost concern in DBT is patient safety. A rescue shock must be administered promptly if the patient remains in fibrillation.

Unlike capture or sensing threshold tests which use a step-down procedure, DFT tests should not be unnecessarily repeated. If a patient can be successfully defibrillated at a relatively low shocking

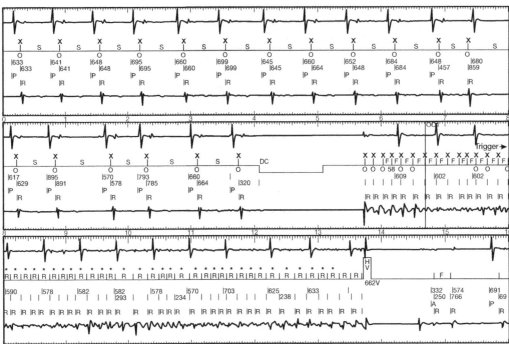

Fig. 5.5 Induction and defibrillation testing. In this example, the patient is successfully induced to ventricular fibrillation (second strip), the device delivers high-energy therapy (third strip), and the patient's sinus rhythm is restored (end of third strip).

energy value, then the physician may terminate the test at that point and not bother to search for an even lower threshold value. There is no universal formula for selecting a defibrillation safety margin. Programmed output settings are based on the clinical experience of the physician. Most devices allow for programming different therapy deliveries, so a patient with a 5 J threshold may be programmed to receive a first shock at 10 J (which would be a 2:1 safety margin), a second at 15 J and a third at maximum energy. However, a patient with a 10 J threshold may be programmed to receive a first shock at 15 J (5 J safety margin, less than 2:1), a second at 20 J and a third at maximum energy.

High DFTs

Of particular concern during DBT is the patient who has a high DFT at implant. Although there is no formal definition of 'high DFT,' as a general rule

it is considered to be any DFT which is within 10 J of the device's maximum delivered energy output. For example, if a manufacturer states that a device has a maximum delivered output of 30 J, then a 20 J or higher threshold value is considered high. Obviously, in such patients, maximum energy shocks are to be programmed, but will they be enough to defibrillate the heart?

Fortunately, there are a few strategies that can be undertaken during DBT to make defibrillation therapy more effective.

One approach is to try a different lead placement, since moving the lead even slightly may reduce the patient's DFT. For some patients, a more elaborate type of lead such as a subcutaneous patch lead or Array-type lead may be required. But before new hardware is introduced to the patient, some other options should be tested, if available. These include changing the tilt value and changing the shocking vector (reversing polarity).

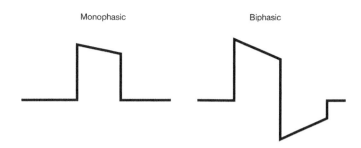

Fig. 5.6 Monophasic and biphasic waveforms. For reasons that are not entirely clear, a monophasic waveform of defibrillation energy is less effective at defibrillating the heart than the biphasic waveform.

Tilt

It was discovered years ago that when high-energy therapy was delivered in a biphasic waveform, it was more effective at defibrillating the heart than the so-called monophasic waveform.[1] A monophasic waveform is defined as a shock waveform delivered in one polarity, that is, traveling only in one direction with respect to the baseline (see Fig. 5.6).

A biphasic waveform typically uses less energy to defibrillate the heart than a monophasic waveform.[2] A biphasic waveform consists of two phases, with the first phase positive, that is, traveling upward from the baseline, and the second phase negative. The second phase is always shorter than or equal to the first phase; the second phase is never longer than the first.

It is unclear as to why biphasic waveforms are so effective.[3] One theory holds that the first phase distorts cell membrane molecules, disturbs ion channels, and leads to continued arrhythmias while the second phase restores cell membrane molecules, leaves the ion channels relatively intact, and terminates arrhythmias. While some older devices relied on the monophasic waveform, today, virtually all ICDs rely on a biphasic waveform. However, to understand the function of tilt – which may be a programmable option to improve defibrillation efficacy – it is important to understand the defibrillating waveform.

Tilt is defined as the percentage drop in voltage on the capacitor from the beginning to the end of each phase over the course of one entire pulse. Based on the waveform, the formula for tilt is $(V1–V2)/V1 \times 100\%$ where V1 is the leading edge and V2 is the trailing edge (see Fig. 5.7).

One study has shown that the most effective tilt values for defibrillating the heart are values between 40% and 65%.[4] This may seem counterintuitive, since a higher tilt corresponds to greater delivered energy. However, it is known that a tilt of 65% is more effective at defibrillating the heart than a tilt value of 80%. But how can clinicians regulate tilt? When it comes to energy delivery, ICDs use either a fixed tilt system or a fixed pulse width system. A fixed tilt system keeps an effective tilt value and delivers the amount of energy programmed, but varies the pulse width as needed to accomplish that goal. Thus, the tilt is fixed, the energy is set, and then based on the impedance values, the ICD automatically changes the pulse width to assure the right amount of programmed energy. This system is used by Medtronic, Guidant, and St Jude Medical.

However, St Jude Medical and earlier Ventritex systems also allow the clinician to select a fixed pulse width system. In such cases, the pulse width is set to a fixed value and the shock energy is programmed in volts. Based on the impedance value, the device changes the tilt setting to assure the proper output.

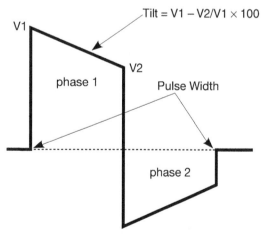

Fig. 5.7 Biphasic waveform with tilt formula. Tilt is defined as the percentage voltage drop between the leading edge and trailing edge of the waveform. This can be calculated as $(V1 – V2)/V1 \times 100\%$.

While a fixed tilt setting is the more common, is available in virtually all ICDs today (and is the default setting of St Jude Medical devices), it may be possible that other devices allow for the programmable option of fixed pulse width. In such cases, the fixed pulse width configuration may provide more effective defibrillation. At any rate, it is definitely an option worth testing in the event that high DFTs are encountered at implant.

Changing the shocking vector and reversing polarity

The shocking vector defines the pathway that defibrillating energy takes through the heart. When a shock is delivered to the heart, the energy must form a circuit from positive pole to negative pole. In conventional defibrillation leads with two coils, there is a coil at the distal end of the right ventricular lead (RV coil) and there is another more proximal coil near the superior vena cava (SVC coil). A shock can make its circuit between RV and SVC coils, allowing for a relatively tight pathway. In such a case, the RV coil is the positive pole, the SVC coil is the negative pole.

For reasons not entirely clear to scientists, changing the pathway of the current through the heart can make defibrillation energy more effective. In such cases, the shocking vector can be reprogrammed so that the energy flows from the RV coil (positive pole) to the device can itself (negative pole). By programming RV-to-can polarity, the shocking vector shifts and widens. This programmable step effectively eliminates the second SVC coil as a pole. This feature is not available in all ICDs, but when it is available, it should be utilized when conducting DBT on patients with high DFTs. It may be that defibrillation efficacy can be improved without the need to increase energy values.

In devices with programmable shocking vectors, the RV coil is typically the positive pole of the circuit (default setting). Programmable polarity allows the clinician to reverse polarity by making the RV coil negative and the SVC coil or the can the positive pole. This change may improve defibrillation efficacy without the need for increasing energy.

The use of these features is limited to those unusual cases when the patient has a high DFT at implant and the clinical team is trying to find ways to enhance therapy delivery.

Concluding the implant procedure

Once the implanting physician is satisfied that the therapy output parameters are appropriate, the implant is nearly over. The physician will place the ICD generator into the pocket and close it up.

The device parameters should be programmed to the appropriate detection, diagnostic, and therapy settings. Bradycardia parameters should be programmed as well. If the patient does not need regular pacing support, it is wise to program very conservative pacing settings. However, if the patient requires pacing, then the appropriate settings should be programmed, including hysteresis, rate response, and mode switching, if available. Once the device is programmed, print out a copy of the programmed settings and measured data for the patient's file. Some physicians have found it useful to print out an extra copy of programmed parameters to give to the patient; the patient can then keep them and pass them along to his or her other doctors or present them to emergency room staff in the event the patient requires interim emergency care.

Paperwork should conclude the procedure, including registering the device and making sure to reserve the patient a copy of his or her temporary ID card and patient manual.

Postoperative care

After the implantation, an ECG should be obtained showing appropriate pacing behavior. A chest X-ray should also be taken post-implant to be used as a baseline for lead placement, in the event that the patient experiences lead complications in the future. In addition, the chest X-ray can verify that the patient is not experiencing any lung problems, pneumothorax, fluid overload, or other potentially dangerous conditions.

The patient will presumably be prescribed a course of antibiotics for the recovery period. A follow-up appointment should be made and, if appropriate, the patient can be given patient literature and contact numbers as well as advice as to what to do in the event of therapy delivery.

References

1   Mouchawar G, Kroll M, Val-Mejias JE. ICD waveform

optimization: a randomized, prospective, pair-sampled multicenter study. *Pacing Clin Electrophysiol* 2000; **23**: 1992–5.

2 Geddes LA, Havel W. Evolution of the optimum bidirectional (biphasic) waveform for defibrillation. *Biomed Instrum Technol* 2000; **34**: 39–54.

3 Mowrey KA, Cheng Y, Tchou PJ, Efimov R. Kinetics of defibrillation shock-induced response: design implications for the optimal defibrillation waveform. *Europace* 2002; **4**: 27–39.

4 Yamanouchi Y, Brewer JE, Donohoo AM *et al*. External exponential biphasic versus monophasic shock waveform: efficacy in ventricular fibrillation of longer duration. *PACE* 1999; **22**: 1481–7.

The nuts and bolts of ICD implant procedures

- ICDs once required a thoracotomy and a hospital stay of several days; today, most systems can be implanted on an outpatient basis in a couple of hours. Transvenous leads and smaller pectoral ICDs in the 1990s made this possible. Today, ICDs are most often implanted in an operating room, cardiac catheterization lab or EP lab.
- ICDs are generally implanted in the upper left pectoral region unless there are compelling reasons (such as a left-handed patient) to use the right region.
- An ICD implant team involves an implanting physician (usually an electrophysiologist or a surgeon), a healthcare professional in charge of anesthesia, a scrub nurse, a circulating nurse, and a representative of the company that manufactures the device.
- A capacitor maintenance charge should be performed prior to implantation to verify that the device is working according to specifications.
- Devices should be implanted before their 'use-before' date on the label. Once the date passes, the device may not have the same longevity as a newer device. The reason for this is that there is some battery current drain even on a device sitting on a shelf (housekeeping current).
- Today, most ICD implants are done under conscious sedation but a general anesthesia may be used in some cases.
- The implanting physician makes a pocket and accesses a vein for inserting the leads in much the same way as is done for pacemaker implantation. The most common venous access is subclavian stick or cephalic cut-down. However, other veins may be used depending on the patient's anatomy and the physician's surgical judgment.
- After leads are placed in the heart, they must be tested for P-waves and R-waves (that is, their ability to sense intrinsic activity). Capture and sensing tests should be performed for pacing.
- A high-voltage lead integrity check should be performed. This delivers a moderately high-voltage therapy to the heart and verifies that the shocking lead is functioning properly.
- Device-based testing (DBT) uses the device to be implanted to help perform defibrillation threshold (DFT) testing to verify that the device will terminate tachyarrhythmias.
- The programmer cannot be sterilized, so place the telemetry wand in a sterile plastic pouch to introduce it into the sterile field.
- Lead impedance values are not programmable but should be carefully checked. If lead impedance values are out of range, it indicates a serious problem with the leads (such as faulty connection, dislodgement, fractured coil, or damaged insulation).
- The DFT defines the lowest amount of energy required to defibrillate the heart. DFT testing may be performed at implant, but is not always done if the implanting physician decides to program the device automatically to maximum settings or feels it is otherwise not warranted.
- If DFT testing is done, fibrillation is induced and then the device tries to terminate it. The device can be used to induce fibrillation (shock-on-T, direct current shocks, programmed stimulation options) and equipment and team should be ready to rescue the patient in the event the device does not defibrillate the patient.
- During DFT testing, the team should verify that the device sensed, detected, and diagnosed

Continued p.36.

Continued.

properly during the episode, that the shock was delivered in a reasonable charge time at an appropriate energy and that it defibrillated the heart. The shocking impedance should also be verified.

- There is no standard formula for safety margin for programming shocking energy values based on a DFT. Most device experts use their best judgment, based on the patient's DFT, the device's capabilities, and how it is going to be programmed. Some physicians will opt to program the device to maximum energy in the first shock; in such cases, DFT testing (which typically regulates less than maximal shocks) may be superfluous.
- High DFTs are defined as those within 10 J of the maximum delivered energy of the device, in other words, DFTs around 20 J. For patients with high DFTs, changing the lead placement, reversing shocking polarity, changing shocking vectors, changing tilt, or even using different lead equipment may make defibrillation more effective, even without increasing actual energy output.
- Tilt is defined as the percentage drop in voltage on the capacitor from the leading edge to the trailing edge of each phase of the biphasic waveform. Although it seems counterintuitive, the most effective tilt settings are 40–65% rather than higher values.
- After the procedure, be sure to give the patient his or her temporary ID card, the patient manual, and specific instructions or contact numbers as to what to do in the event of therapy delivery. Some clinics print out an extra copy of the device's programmed parameters for the patient to take to his or her next physician, in the event that interim care is required.

CHAPTER 6

Sensing

Sensing in implantable pacemakers and defibrillators refers to the device's ability to pick up intrinsic signals from the heart and interpret them properly, in such a way that allows the device to respond appropriately. A pacemaker (or the pacemaker function within a defibrillator) that detects a properly timed, intrinsic ventricular depolarization receives that information, recognizes it as a sensed ventricular event and, on the basis of that information, withholds a ventricular output pulse. Clinicians experienced in pacemaker therapy are used to sensitivity settings programmed as fixed values.

ICD sensing created a challenge for both clinicians and engineers because there is a wide variation in the size of signals the average patient might experience. While a normal ventricular signal might be fairly large and stable, ventricular tachyarrhythmias, in particular ventricular fibrillation (VF), are often characterized by relatively low amplitude ventricular signals. Thus, an ICD has to be especially sensitive or it risks missing sensing those signals. Yet if sensitivity was set in such a way that such small amplitude signals could be reliably recognized by the ICD, there is a good chance that other low amplitude signals – such as T-waves, far-field signals, and myopotentials – would also get detected.

When it comes to sensing, a device needs to be sensitive enough to pick up those signals it needs to recognize. If it is not sensitive enough, those signals will get missed and the device will not respond. This phenomenon is called 'undersensing,' and a good way to think of it is that for bradycardia therapy, undersensing = overpacing. When a device undersenses, most systems will end up pacing inappropriately.

On the other hand, a device can be set in such a way that it is sensitive enough to pick up the signals it needs to recognize, but it may be so sensitive that it picks up a lot of other noise as well. This phenomenon is called 'oversensing' and it leads to underpacing, that is, the system will be inhibited more than it ought to be because it is seeing inappropriate signals and counting them as appropriate signals.

There was probably no greater technological hurdle in merging pacing function to defibrillation than figuring out how to manage sensing. Pacemakers need to sense reliably in order to pace appropriately, but sensing in the presence of variable-amplitude tachyarrhythmic signals was complicated. That challenge was met with sophisticated sensing algorithms for ICDs which allow for automatic, dynamic sensitivity setting adjustments.

The theory behind all automatic sensing systems is that signal amplitudes are processed and the sensitivity setting is based on the most recently sensed amplitudes. Refractory periods are launched with sensing but when they time out, it is possible for lower amplitude signals to break through and reset the sensitivity; this might occur when a patient suddenly goes into VF. On the other hand, the presence of large, well-defined ventricular activity resets the sensitivity in such a way that reliably filters out T-waves and interference.

The major ICD manufacturers all offer variations on automatic, dynamically adjusting sensitivity. While specifics will vary by manufacturer and device, the same general principles apply. This book will discuss the St Jude Medical algorithm in detail.

The intracardiac electrogram provides the best representation of the signals that an ICD 'sees,' but the tracing that appears on the programmer screen has been processed from raw data. The raw signal enters the system and gets filtered in such a way that the T-wave portion is minimized, noise is reduced, and any far-field signals are filtered out. This raw signal has positive and negative deflections. For the purposes of the Auto Sensitivity algorithm, the signal is digitally rectified (electronically corrected) in such a way that it is all positive. This digitally modified signal is the one used for the sensing algorithm (see Fig. 6.1).

When a ventricular signal is sensed, it begins a sensed refractory period. During this sensed refractory period, the ICD measures the peak of the maximum amplitude that occurs during that sensed refractory period window. This does not terminate the sensed refractory period or reset the rate; it simply establishes a peak signal amplitude for that particular complex (see Fig. 6.2).

This peak amplitude value is stored and used to determine a function called Threshold Start. When the sensed refractory period expires, the sensitivity

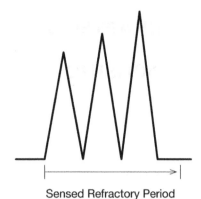

Sensed Refractory Period

Fig. 6.2 Peak amplitude measurement during sensed refractory period. At the point at which a signal is sensed, it launches a sensed refractory period timing cycle. The signal with the highest peak during this sensed refractory period timing cycle is recorded and remembered by the ICD as the peak amplitude of that cycle. (The peak amplitude does not reset the timer.)

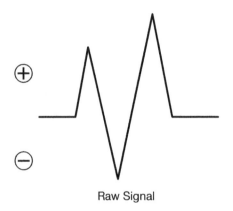

Raw Signal

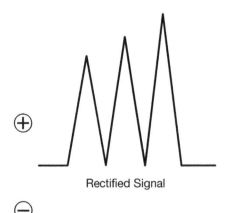

Rectified Signal

Fig. 6.1 Raw signal and digitally rectified signal. The raw signal has positive and negative deflections. It is filtered, the T-wave is minimized, noise and far-field signals are reduced, and the entire signal is digitally rectified in such a way that all deflections are now positive.

is set to the value of Threshold Start. Threshold Start is described as a percentage of the maximum peak amplitude of the previous cycle. Nominally, Threshold Start is set at 50% but other values can be programmed. The idea is that Threshold Start defines how the sensitivity setting for the next cardiac cycle will be set at the start. There is a linear decline from Threshold Start down to the maximum sensitivity setting, but the Threshold Start value determines where the slope begins (see Figs 6.3 and 6.4).

Thus, Auto Sensitivity assesses a peak amplitude during each sensed refractory period, uses this to determine a Threshold Start value, and creates a sensitivity 'window' that changes as the patient's own intrinsic activity changes. This helps the device to sense small or erratically sized signals, which can be common during ventricular tachyarrhythmias (see Fig. 6.5).

It is always a good idea to refer to the device manual or other product specifications to understand all of the parameter settings. The Threshold Start in Auto Sensitivity in current St Jude Medical devices is programmed nominally to 50% for native R-waves between 2 and 6 mV. For large R-waves, over 6 mV, the Threshold Start value caps at 3 mV (in other words, if a peak amplitude is 7 mV, the Threshold Start at 50% does not exceed 3.0 mV). Likewise, if an R-wave is < 2 mV, the Threshold Start at 50% does not fall below 1.0 mV.

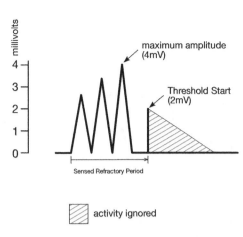

Fig. 6.3 Threshold Start. When the ventricular signal was sensed, it launched the sensed refractory period, during which the ICD recorded the peak amplitude that occurred (4 mV). When the sensed refractory period timed out, it launched Auto Sensitivity. The new sensitivity setting was set at 50% of the peak amplitude or 2 mV. From that point, there was a linear decay of sensitivity down to maximum sensitivity. The shaded area shows the area in which signals would be ignored.

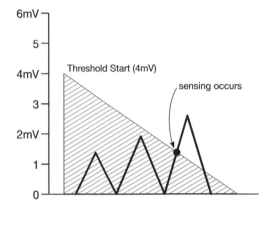

Fig. 6.4 Activity ignored. In this close-up of the area defined by the Threshold Start down to the maximum sensitivity value, the ICD ignores signals entirely in the shaded area, such as the first two waves. However, a signal large enough to break out of the shaded area (third signal) would be sensed.

An ICD also uses automatic sensitivity algorithms for atrial sensing. The Threshold Start is set nominally to 50% for atrial sensing in St Jude Medical devices for peak amplitudes between 0.6 mV and 3.0 mV. If a P-wave is > 3.0 mV, the Threshold Start does not exceed 1.5 mV, and if it is < 0.6 mV, the Threshold Start is never lower than 0.3 mV.

In Auto Sensitivity, the normal decay of the sensitivity 'triangle' is linear with about 1 mV decay every 312 ms on the ventricular channel and 0.5 mV decay every 312 ms on the atrial channel. Yet in some cases, a clinician may feel that the device needs to be less sensitive than even that. This may occur when there is a lot of myopotential noise, large T-waves, electromagnetic interference or other far-field signals. In such cases, the clinician can program a feature called the Decay Delay (see Fig. 6.6). This is a timing parameter (programmable in milliseconds) that holds the Threshold Start value for the programmed amount of time before the downward decay slope begins. This feature is not something that is routinely programmed for the average patient, so St Jude Medical ICDs are shipped with this parameter set to the nominal value of 0. However, Decay Delay can help make ICDs less likely to sense inappropriate signals.

The decay is a linear decline which stops when it hits the maximum sensitivity setting (which is sort of a floor or baseline for sensitivity) or whenever the next signal is sensed. Maximum sensitivity is a value many clinicians know from pacemakers, but it has a somewhat different function in ICDs. In pacemakers, maximum sensitivity defines the highest sensitivity setting (that is, the lowest mV value) that the device can reliably sense.

Dual-chamber ICDs require clinicians to program three independent maximum sensitivity settings. The first two relate to the pacemaker function of the device: there is a maximum sensitivity setting for the atrial channel (nominally 0.2 mV) and for the ventricular channel (nominally 0.3 mV). This is the most sensitive setting of the device. The Thresh-

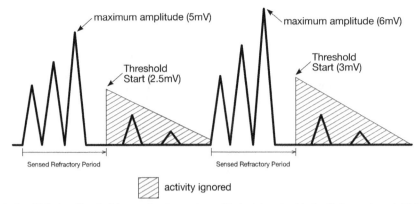

Fig. 6.5 Auto Sensitivity in action. In this complex, the peak amplitude determined in the first complex establishes the Threshold Start used when the sensed refractory period expires. The next signal is sensed, initiates the sensed refractory period timing cycle, and creates a new value for Threshold Start. In this way, sensitivity adjusts with the patient's intrinsic signals.

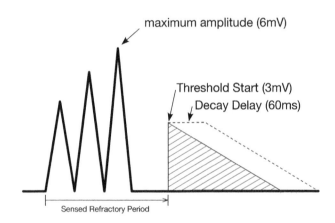

Fig. 6.6 Decay Delay. The peak amplitude measured during the sensed refractory period is 3 mV, and at the 50% Threshold Start value, this sets the sensitivity 'triangle' for the next cycle at 1.5 mV. With a 60 ms Decay Delay programmed, the 1.5 mV value is maintained for 60 ms before the linear decay begins. The dotted lines show how the sensitivity would have decayed with a nominal Decay Delay of 60 ms.

old Start and other related parameters allow the device to be temporarily less sensitive in order to avoid sensing small but inappropriate signals, such as the T-wave or other noise. But the Threshold Start always decays toward the maximum sensitivity value, which makes the device sensitive to even very small signals.

The defibrillator portion of the ICD also requires the setting of a maximum sensitivity value, which in the current generation of St Jude Medical devices is 0.3 mV in the device as shipped. (Consult with product literature for the specifics about a particular ICD. There can be considerable variation in specifications, even from a single manufacturer.) This relatively low mV setting (or high sensitivity) assures that low amplitude ventricular fibrillation signals can be detected, but the other

parameters provide reasonable assurance that most T-waves and other inappropriate signals will get blocked.

Whenever a signal crosses a 'sensitivity boundary' outside of the sensed refactory period, the ICD sees that as a sensed event. It is possible for the ICD to sense an event on the upward or downward slope of a wave. A sensed event launches a new sensed refractory period timing cycle (see Fig. 6.7).

A dual-chamber ICD also requires atrial sensing, and it is here that fixed sensitivity settings (similar to pacemakers) can be used, or an automatic algorithm can be applied. A fixed sensitivity value can work in dual-chamber ICD patients when they have relatively uniform atrial signals. Since patients are not rescued from atrial arrhythmias by the ICD, there is less danger in missing or inappropriately sensing atrial

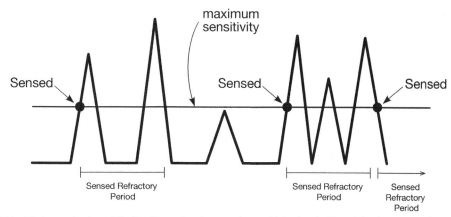

Fig. 6.7 Ventricular sensing in an ICD. Any time a signal crosses the sensitivity threshold outside of a sensed refractory period, the ICD counts it as a sensed event. This resets the sensed refractory timing cycle. Note that an event can be sensed on the upstroke or downstroke of a given signal.

signals. For this reason, it may be appropriate to rely on a fixed atrial sensitivity value for atrial sensing. However, an automatic sensitivity algorithm is available and many clinicians prefer this dynamic and automatically self-adjusting algorithm.

Thus far, the sensitivity information in this chapter relates to sensing intrinsic cardiac activity. For an ICD, nothing is more crucial than being able to detect dangerous ventricular arrhythmias. However, most dual-chamber ICDs will also have to recognize and respond to paced activity as well. When a timing cycle expires and an output pulse is delivered to either the atrium or ventricle, the chamber depolarizes milliseconds before the device senses that a depolarization is occurring. For this reason, most ICDs use slightly different refractory period timing cycles depending on whether the initiating event was sensed or paced. A post-pace refractory period is typically shorter. The Threshold Start value still applies, but it sets itself automatically.

The ventricular post-pace Threshold Start is based on the notion that the QT interval will shorten progressively as the paced rate increases. Thus, as the paced rate gets faster, the Threshold Start value will get lower (and the Decay Delay, if programmed, will shorten). The overall impact of these settings is that when pacing at a higher rate, the ICD becomes more sensitive. Remember that ventricular tachyarrhythmias are often low amplitude or erratic amplitude signals. When the ICD starts pacing, particularly at fairly rapid rates, the device becomes more sensitive to smaller amplitude signals.

These functions all relate to sensing, which is the proper interpretation of intrinsic cardiac activity so that the device can respond appropriately. This is not to be confused with 'detection,' which refers to the ICD's ability to recognize certain types of arrhythmias and respond appropriately. Both sensing and detection rely on sensitivity but sensing helps guide pacing function while detection controls therapy delivery (shocks).

The nuts and bolts of sensing

- Sensing was an engineering challenge to dual-chamber ICD development, because ICDs need to be able to sense potentially low amplitude ventricular tachyarrhythmias but not oversense T-waves, far-field signals, or noise.
- The intracardiac electrogram (IEGM) is the most reliable way to see what the ICD sees.
- For an IEGM, the raw intracardiac signal is taken, filtered, processed, and digitally rectified in order for the device to better evaluate it.
- Oversensing = underpacing and undersensing = overpacing.
- Dual-chamber ICDs rely on dynamically adjusting sensitivity algorithms.
- When an event is sensed, it launches a sensed refractory period. When a paced event is sensed, it launches a post-pace refractory period, which is a little bit shorter than the sensed refractory period.
- The Threshold Start sets sensitivity at each complex based on the peak amplitude of the preceding complex (nominally 50%, so a 5 mV peak amplitude results in a 2.5 mV Threshold Start). This allows for dynamic sensitivity settings.
- The maximum sensitivity setting is the highest sensitivity (or lowest mV value) at which the device will sense.
- The Threshold Start makes the device temporarily less sensitive right after a refractory period expires. The Threshold Start decays linearly down to the maximum sensitivity rate.
- Most dual-chamber ICDs require the clinician to program three separate maximum sensitivity settings: one for the atrial pacing channel, one for the ventricular pacing channel, and one for the ventricular ICD channel.
- An innovative feature from St Jude Medical called Decay Delay allows the device to be temporarily less sensitive when a sensed refractory period expires for a programmable amount of time. This can help fine-tune sensing for some patients.
- Sensing occurs whenever a waveform 'breaks through' a sensitivity boundary outside of a refractory period. Sensing may occur on the upstroke or downstroke of a wave.
- A dual-chamber ICD can use a fixed sensitivity setting on the atrial channel, but not on the ventricular channel. Even on the atrial channel, many clinicians will prefer an automatically adjusting sensitivity algorithm.
- Different devices (and even different models from the same manufacturer) may offer different algorithms and specifics for sensitivity but they are all based on the principle of automatically adjusting the ICD's sensitivity on a beat by beat basis.

CHAPTER 7

Arrhythmia detection

In order for an ICD to deliver therapy for specific tachyarrhythmias, it needs a reliable method to sort out arrhythmias, group them by categories, and make a determination as to when therapy delivery is mandated. These various steps are all part of the arrhythmia detection function of an ICD and depend on the sensing parameter settings of the device. If the ICD is undersensing, there is a risk that important signals (which might have led to therapy delivery) will drop out and not be counted. If the ICD is oversensing, it is possible that the ICD will double-count some events or sense T-waves, both of which could lead to inaccurately high counts, possibly resulting in inappropriate therapy delivery.

Since proper therapy delivery can literally be a matter of life and death, the detection algorithms in ICDs must have a high sensitivity for detecting the ventricular tachyarrhythmias. The ICD uses information from the intracardiac electrogram (IEGM) for gathering the information it will use to categorize the heart rhythm. Most devices have three broad detection categories defined by rate: normal sinus rhythm (NSR), ventricular tachyarrhythmias, and ventricular fibrillation (VF) (see Table 7.1). While these rhythms are defined by rate, the device actually looks at the corresponding cycle lengths or millisecond (ms) intervals to make its determinations.

Most ICDS today offer tiered therapy, meaning that there are different electrical therapies for different types of detected arrhythmias. These types of therapies include:

- Antitachycardia pacing (ATP) or low-voltage patterned stimulation.
- Cardioversion or low-energy shocks.
- Defibrillation or high-energy shocks.

While some particularly dangerous and aggressive tachyarrhythmias may require high-energy defibrillation to convert, many slower or otherwise less aggressive rhythm disorders may respond favorably to lower energy treatments. By using ATP or lower energy cardioverting shocks, the device saves energy and the patient is not subjected to a full output shock, but the rhythm disorder is still terminated.

In order to program how rhythm disorders are to be defined and which type of therapy to apply to which rhythm disorders, the clinician must program the device into detection zones (sometimes called the device configuration). A detection zone sets up rate-based (interval) definitions for various cardiac rhythms.

Defib Only

For Defib Only, the device is programmed so that it recognizes only two types of rhythms: NSR, which it does not treat, and VF, which requires therapy delivery in the form of a high-energy shock. While settings can be fine-tuned, NSR would generally fall in the range of any rate below 200 bpm. VF would be any rate above 200 bpm. When VF is detected, the device delivers a high-energy shock. When programming the cut-off values for these rate categories, it is important to recognize that these are not

Table 7.1 How the ICD defines rhythms

Rhythm category	Rate	Interval
Normal sinus rhythm (NSR)	60–100 bpm	1000 ms to 600 ms
Ventricular tachycardia (VT)	100–200 bpm	600 ms to 300 ms
Ventricular fibrillation (VF)	200–400 bpm	400 ms to 250 ms

Defib with Single Tach Zone

In this configuration, the device recognizes three rhythms: NSR, which it does not treat; Tach A, which it treats with ATP or cardioversion; and VF, which requires delivery of a high-energy shock. While the rates can be adjusted, NSR might be anything below 120 bpm, Tach A could be anything between 120 and 200 bpm, and VF might be everything above 200 bpm. If the device were configured in this manner, when an arrhythmia of 170 bpm was detected, the device would respond with ATP or low-energy shocks. If the device detected a ventricular rhythm of 300 bpm, it would not bother with ATP or low-energy shocks, but it would immediately deliver high-energy therapy.

Defib with Tach A and Tach B

In this configuration, the clinician can set up four zones: NSR, Tach A, Tach B, and VF. Tach A would be the slower range of ventricular tachycardia (VT), while Tach B would be the higher range of VT. An example of this configuration might be to define NSR as anything below 120 bpm, Tach A (slow VT) to be anything between 120 and 160 bpm, Tach B (faster VT) would fall between 160 and 200 bpm, and VF would be any ventricular rhythm above 200 bpm (see Tables 7.2 and 7.3).

The ICD measures intervals or cycle lengths from the intracardiac electrogram. Interval can be defined as the time in milliseconds between any two consecutive ventricular events (either sensed or paced).

Rather than viewing intervals in isolation, the ICD may use a process known as 'interval averaging' to smooth out the potential bumps that might be introduced if each interval were counted in isolation. (For example, a premature ventricular contraction or PVC might fall into the VF range rather than being viewed in its proper context as an unusual single event.) In the interval averaging process, the device counts an interval by measuring the present interval and then taking the three prior intervals and dividing by four. In this way, the rate variations that might be introduced with PVCs or other occasional events do not unduly influence detection schemes (see Fig. 7.1).

The ICD next has to decide how to count (and where to categorize) the intervals. If the *current in-*

Table 7.2 ICD configurations

Configuration	Zones	Suitability
Defib Only	Sinus (< 200 bpm)	When patient would not be likely respond to ATP or
	Fib (> 200 bpm)	cardioversion
Defib with Single Tach Zone	Sinus (< 120 bpm)	When patient has stable VTs that respond to ATP or
	Tach A (120–200 bpm)	cardioversion
	Fib (> 200 bpm)	
Defib with Tach A and Tach B	Sinus (< 120 bpm)	When patients have different types of VTs that are stable
	Tach A (120–160 bpm)	and respond to ATP or cardioversion (e.g. fast VT and slow
	Tach B (160–200 bpm)	VT requiring treatment)
	Fib (> 200 bpm)	

Table 7.3 Zone programmability

Zone	Rate	Intervals	Programmable steps
Single Tach Zone	102–200 bpm	590 ms to 300 ms	5 ms
Tach A	102–194 bpm	590 ms to 310 ms	5 ms
Tach B	109–214 bpm	550 ms to 280 ms	5 ms
Fib	150–240 bpm	590 ms to 300 ms	10 ms

Note that this information is based on certain St Jude Medical ICDs and may vary for other devices. Always refer to the physician's manual for information specific to any given device.

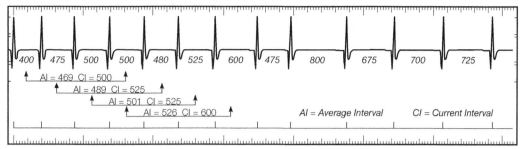

Fig. 7.1 Interval averaging. When the fourth interval (500 ms) is measured, the device measures that interval and the preceding three intervals (400 + 475 + 500 + 500 = 1875) then divides by four (468.75) and reports that number, in this case rounded up, as the interval (469).

terval and the *average interval* fall into the same category (for example, Tach A), the interval is counted (or 'binned') in that rate zone. However, sometimes the current interval and the average interval fall into two different zones. When that occurs, the interval is binned in the faster zone, because the ICD is set up to err on the side of patient safety. In the event that either the current interval or the average interval is classified as NSR, then it is binned as sinus, even though sinus rhythm does not ever result in therapy delivery.

In order to prevent an occasional single-beat rhythm variation from resulting in therapy delivery, the ICD is set up so that if only one of the two (current interval or average interval) is sinus, the interval is not counted at all. (See Tables 7.4 and 7.5.)

Table 7.4 Binning decisions when the ICD is set to Defib Only

Current interval	Average interval	Bin decision
Sinus	Sinus	Sinus
Fib	Sinus	Not binned
Sinus	Fib	Not binned
Fib	Fib	Fib

Table 7.5 Binning decisions when the ICD is configured with a single tach zone

Current interval	Average interval	Bin decision
Sinus	Sinus	Sinus
Tach	Tach	Tach
Fib	Fib	Fib
Tach	Sinus	Not binned
Fib	Sinus	Not binned
Fib	Tach	Fib
Tach	Fib	Fib

Binning is a constant process that involves every single recorded interval. The status of the counting process can be monitored on the programmer's IEGM.

The ICD will not deliver therapy until the device can make a diagnosis of a rhythm disorder based on interval data in the bins. In simplistic terms, the ICD diagnoses a rhythm disorder when it counts enough intervals in that particular rate bin. The device counts constantly and keeps intervals in all bins; the first bin to reach the critical mass necessary to establish the diagnosis initiates the sequence of events that will culminate in therapy delivery (and 'shuts off' the other bins).

In all tach zones (whether one or Tach A/Tach B), the clinician has the option of programming the number of intervals required for a diagnosis to be made, usually within a broad range (for example, 6 to 100 intervals). In many St Jude Medical ICDs, the nominal setting is 12 intervals.

For fibrillation, a much more serious arrhythmia, the range is much tighter. While actual ranges may vary by manufacturer, a typical range would be 8 intervals for fast fib detection, 16 for slow fib detection, and 12 as a nominal or default setting.

The intervals do not have to be consecutive to establish a diagnosis, but must fall within a range (for example 12 events, in any order, in a consecutive series of 16 events). This method allows for the fact that a rhythm disorder does not always start consistently and that very high-rate activity is often punctuated by slower or even normal range beats (see Fig. 7.2).

The intracardiac electrogram as seen on the programmer captures what occurs during arrhythmia detection. The sequence of consecutive events is marked out along with cycles that count toward

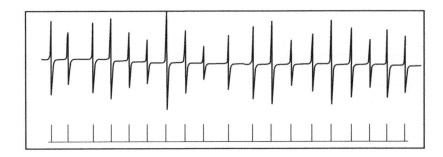

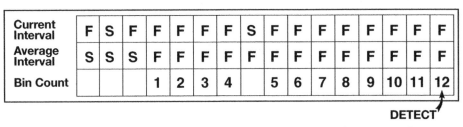

Current Interval	F	S	F	F	F	F	F	S	F	F	F	F	F	F	F	F
Average Interval	S	S	S	F	F	F	F	F	F	F	F	F	F	F	F	F
Bin Count				1	2	3	4		5	6	7	8	9	10	11	12

DETECT

Fig. 7.2 Binning. In this chart, F stands for Fib and S is Sinus. When the device binned 12 fib events out of a consecutive 16 event run, the device would 'detect' fibrillation.

meeting interval criteria for the particular rhythm disorder (see Fig. 7.3).

Binning for tachycardia is accomplished in the same way. The device counts intervals until detection criteria are met and a diagnosis can be made (see Fig. 7.4).

One of the design challenges in creating a functional ICD involved having the device monitor whether or not a therapy delivery was sufficient to convert the rhythm disorder and if a second therapy delivery might be required. To accomplish this, ICDs employ a technique known as 'redetection,' which allows the device to check on a rhythm post-shock and determine if additional therapy might be needed.

Redetection requires the ICD to bin a programmable number of sinus intervals following therapy delivery. While the number of sinus intervals required will vary by device, it is typically in the range of three to seven with a nominal setting of five. In some instances, the ICD will determine that the arrhythmia continues even after therapy has been delivered. In those cases, a certain number of intervals must be binned before the device will deliver another therapy. Fib redetection is fixed at 6 intervals in St Jude Medical devices, but tachycardia redetection may be programmed in a range from typically 6 to 20 intervals with a nominal value of 6 (see Figs 7.5 and 7.6).

Redetection is a very important function of an ICD. The clinician has certain programming options in terms of determining how to define the reestablishment of sinus rhythm (in terms of number of sinus events) or resumption of tachycardia. Since VF is such a serious rhythm disorder, the redetection criterion is fixed at six intervals, simply because of the potentially disastrous consequences of allowing a patient to remain too long in a fibrillatory state.

When an arrhythmia is redetected after a less aggressive therapy delivery, the next arrhythmia may be treated with a progressively more aggressive approach. For example, if VT is redetected after ATP is administered, the next therapy may be a low-energy shock or even a high-energy shock. On the other hand, if the patient tolerates VT well and generally responds to ATP, a clinician might want to program the device to treat the VT several times with ATP before progressing to more aggressive, higher energy options.

There are additional parameters involved in arrhythmia detection which will be discussed in later chapters. These special features are Maximum Time to Diagnosis (MTD) and Maximum Time to Fib (MTF).

Besides these functions, devices can also be configured with Defib Off. This means that the defibrillation function of the ICD is temporarily deactivated

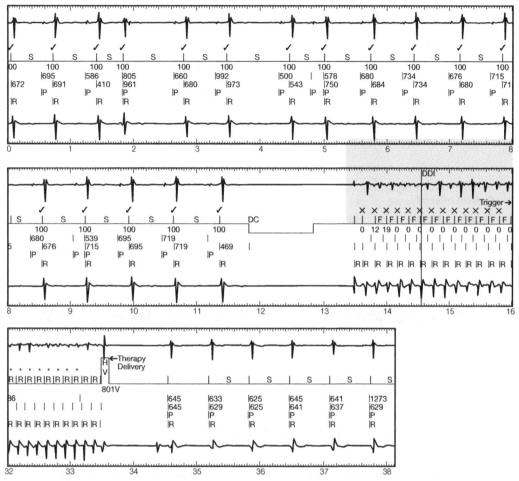

Fig. 7.3 IEGM detection. The device notices Fib Intervals (marked F in the shaded area in the second strip) and counts out the necessary string of consecutive intervals (in this case, 12 out of 13). This satisfies the detection criteria and the device diagnoses fib and prepares for therapy delivery, which appears on the electrogram as HV (high-voltage shock) in the bottom strip. The R events that occur after diagnosis and before the shock are intrinsic events that occur before the device can deliver therapy. After therapy, normal cardiac activity is restored.

so that no high-voltage therapy delivery can occur. While programming Defib Off is an unusual occurrence, it occasionally becomes necessary. Examples of situations where programming defibrillation off might be useful include:

- Patient is undergoing surgery involving electrocautery (shocks during delicate surgery can be disastrous);
- Patient is experiencing many inappropriate shocks;
- Patient is near death and elects to turn the device off.

In most instances, the decision to turn off the device's defibrillating function is for a specific purpose. Often Defib Off is used for only a limited time; defibrillation will soon be turned back on. Restoring previously programmed parameters can usually be accomplished in a one-button ('Restore Parameters') or otherwise simple programming step. The device stores the previously programmed settings in the *memory of the device* (not the memory of the programmer), so it is usually fairly simple to restore previously programmed settings. At that point, settings can be adjusted further, if desired.

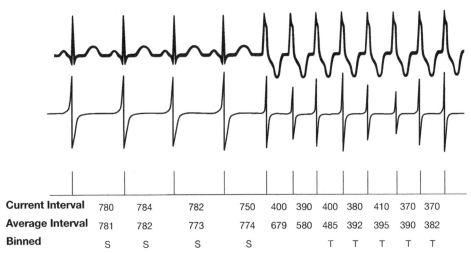

	Current Interval	780	784	782	750	400	390	400	380	410	370	370
	Average Interval	781	782	773	774	679	580	485	392	395	390	382
	Binned	S	S	S	S		T	T	T	T	T

Fig. 7.4 Binning for VT. In this series, the current interval and average interval are measured with events binned as sinus (S), tachycardia (T) or not binned at all (when either current interval or average interval – but not both – is sinus).

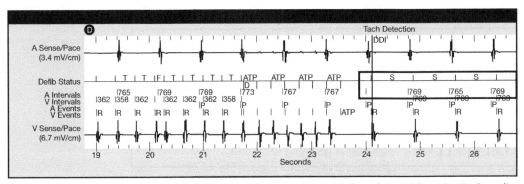

Fig. 7.5 Tachy redetection. In this intracardiac electrogram, the device detected tachycardia and delivered antitachycardia pacing (ATP) therapy, followed by sinus activity. The device was programmed so that three sinus events post-therapy established that therapy was effective and sinus rate restored.

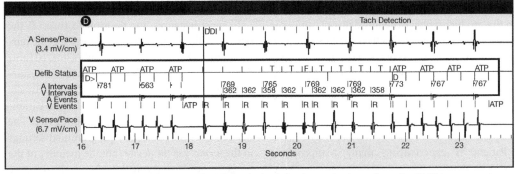

Fig. 7.6 Repeated ATP after tachy redetection. The ICD begins by delivering antitachycardia pacing (ATP) in response to a diagnosed VT. The device was programmed so that six intervals of tach (T) or fib (F) post-therapy established the therapy as ineffective. In this case, the arrhythmia was redetected and a new round of ATP was administered. The decision as to what therapy to apply following arrhythmia redetection can be programmed by the clinician.

The nuts and bolts of arrhythmia detection

- The ICD diagnoses rhythm disorders by counting intervals on the intracardiac electrogram. This is a rate-based detection scheme that can be adjusted to meet the individual patient's needs by programming.
- The ICD counts the current interval as one value and then the average of the current interval and the preceding three intervals. If these events fall into the same category, the event is binned in that category. If one but not both (that is either the current interval or the average interval) is sinus, the interval is not counted. If both events are tachycardia or fibrillation but not in the same category, the interval is binned in the higher category.
- The ICD diagnoses an arrhythmia when a sufficient (and programmable) number of events in an event sequence are binned. This is usually stated in an 'X out of Y' pattern, such as 12 out of 16 intervals.
- ICDs can be configured as Defib Only (recognizing only the rate categories of sinus or fib), Defib with Single Tach (recognizing only the rate categories of sinus, Tach A, or fib) or Defib with Tach A and Tach B (recognizing sinus, Tach A or slow VT, Tach B or fast VT, and fib).
- Different detection schemes and therapies can be programmed for different categories. For example, ATP may be appropriate treatment for slow VT.
- After therapy is delivered, the ICD monitors the next intervals to redetect sinus rate (which means the therapy worked) or redetect the arrhythmia (which results in resumed therapy).

CHAPTER 8

Arrhythmia therapy

ICD therapy is rescue. The goal of ICD therapy is not to alleviate symptoms or enhance well-being or try to improve the patient's underlying condition: it is to rescue the patient from a potentially life-threatening ventricular arrhythmia. When it comes to therapy delivery in an ICD, it can literally be a matter of life and death.

ICDs offer three main categories and two types of therapy: **high-energy** (sometimes called high-voltage) shocks or cardioversion, and **antitachycardia pacing (ATP)**. High-energy shocks and cardioversion are really the same type of therapy: a large amount of electrical energy is sent to the heart to defibrillate it. In the clinical setting, defibrillation is performed using higher energy levels than cardioversion. In the world of implantable devices, cardioversion refers to a shock delivered to terminate a tachycardia, while defibrillation refers to a shock delivered to terminate fibrillation. As a rule of thumb, cardioversion usually involves an output of around 2–15 joules (J), while defibrillation is greater than 15 J. However, in device therapy, defibrillation therapy and cardioversion may actually involve the same amount of energy: the difference is the arrhythmia they are trying to terminate.

ATP uses patterned stimulation at low-voltage levels (typical pacemaker outputs) to terminate ventricular tachyarrhythmia. While most modern ICDs have programmable ATP options, in clinical practice, these options are not always enabled. Older or simple ICDs may not offer ATP.

High-voltage therapy

The great challenge to the design of the ICD was to create a device small enough and safe enough to implant under the skin that was capable of delivering a massive amount of energy (700–800 V or 30–36

J) very quickly. Since ventricular tachyarrhythmias can start suddenly and may be lethal in a matter of minutes, the device had to be able to identify and diagnose a dangerous arrhythmia and then deliver high-voltage therapy in a matter of seconds. Since the typical battery size for an implantable device is about 3.2 V, the challenge seemed more than just daunting. It seemed impossible. How could such a small battery deliver so much energy so quickly?

The answer came in the form of an electronic component known as a capacitor. Developed originally for use in flash photography, capacitors act as high-voltage storage tanks. The battery can 'pump' energy into the capacitor, which holds it until it reaches a predetermined capacity. At that point, the capacitor 'unloads' all of the stored energy in one bolus. Thus, a 3.2 V battery can fill a capacitor to the point that it contains enough energy (700 V) to defibrillate the heart.

Capacitors are some of the largest individual components in an ICD, larger than even the battery. Capacitors are made of two aluminum sheets separated by an oxide dielectric. This dielectric component starts to decay and deform over time if it is not periodically charged to capacity. Deformed capacitors may allow some current stored in the capacitor to leak out, resulting in longer-than-normal charge times to reach defibrillation energy. This can affect device capacitance, which is defined as the capacity of the capacitor.

Fortunately, the easy way to avoid capacitor deformation is to perform a step called 'reforming' or capacitor reformation. Most modern ICDs reform their capacitors automatically, so no clinician intervention is required. However, some older devices and specific types of ICDs may require the clinician to program capacitor maintenance (which may be done in a programming session or programmed to occur automatically at a later time). ICDs with automatic capacitor maintenance use a schedule based on battery voltage and self-adjust as needed.

During capacitor reformation, the device charges to full capacity and then allows that charge to bleed off, that is, to dissipate gradually and harmlessly. When an ICD offers automatic capacitor maintenance, the patient will not be aware of this action; it causes no pain or unusual sensations.

High-voltage shocks are described in volts and in joules. Although both are commonly used expressions, they are actually different units of measure. Voltage refers to an electromotive force as measured in the difference in potentials (the force in one thing versus the force in another). References to voltage are frequently made for household appliances, the action potential of the heart, and battery chemistry. Joules are a unit of energy (specifically the amount of energy it takes to do the work by a force of one Newton acting through a distance of one meter). Most clinicians find it more helpful to talk about defibrillation energy in terms of joules, which measure energy, rather than voltage. Note that there is no direct conversion formula for translating volts into joules precisely and vice versa; factors such as impedance affect the equation.

Defibrillation or cardioversion therapy involves the application of a single high-energy output to the heart. The amount of energy in the shock can be programmed. Clinical considerations as to the amount of energy to program for a therapy delivery involve several factors:

- What is the patient's defibrillation threshold (if known)?
- Is the shock intended to terminate a nonlethal ventricular tachycardia or a life-threatening ventricular tachyarrhythmia?
- Does the patient respond well to lower energy shocks?

The defibrillation threshold (DFT) is defined as the amount of energy required to reliably defibrillate the heart. During implantation, the physician may elect to perform DFT testing, in which ventricular fibrillation is induced and then terminated by the device in a step-down sequence to find the minimum reliable level of energy needed to achieve defibrillation. Since DFT testing involves inducing potentially fatal ventricular fibrillation several times, it can be a difficult, nerve-wracking step of the procedure. It also almost always requires the patient to be under deep sedation or even general anesthesia. Today, some ICD implanters forego DFT testing at implant and program the device to the highest output settings.

Obviously, if the patient's DFT is known and is fairly low, it may not be necessary to program the highest level of energy. ICDs allow the clinician to program multiple therapy deliveries in a step-up sequence, that is, a lower energy shock first, followed by a more aggressive shock and perhaps followed by a maximum shock. This approach requires careful clinical consideration, since if the first shocks do not work, the patient spends an unnecessarily long period of time in a dangerous arrhythmic state.

One reason for programming a lower energy shock might be to terminate an arrhythmia that occurs in a tach zone, rather than in the fib zone. For instance, if the patient is prone to both ventricular fibrillation (VF) as well as hemodynamically stable ventricular tachycardia (VT), setting up a tach zone for the VT allows the clinician to program a therapy that will be administered when the device diagnoses VT as opposed to VF. In such instances, it may be useful to program smaller shocks for this type of arrhythmia, particularly if there is some documentation that shows the patient had previously responded well to lower energy shocks for such arrhythmias. Lower energy shocks spare ICD battery life (high-energy shocks drain the battery) and are often more tolerable for the patient. If it is not necessary to use the highest energy shocks to terminate a stable VT, there is good reason for the clinician to consider a tiered therapeutic strategy.

In actual practice, many clinicians program ICDs to the highest levels of energy output for therapy. The patient may not have undergone DFT testing at implant, may have no documented history of response to shocks at varying degrees of energy, and may not be hemodynamically stable when the device diagnoses an arrhythmia – all of which are good reasons to get powerful therapy fast.

Another consideration involves the DFT itself. One reason many implanters have chosen to forego DFT testing is the fact that DFTs are not constant values.[1] They vary with many factors, including time, disease progression, and drug interactions.[2] Since most ICD patients have heart disease (often multiple conditions) and are on pharmacological therapy for their heart and possibly other conditions, the things that can most affect DFTs seem to describe ICD patients! Many forms of heart disease are progressive, which means that the patient's heart is going to change over time. Unfortunately, changes in DFT levels can be clinically silent. There is simply no way of knowing if the patient's DFT at implant is still the same a year later without subjecting the patient to a new round of DFT tests. As a result, there is good reason for clinicians to program highest energy shocks, particularly in response to the most dangerous forms of ventricular tachyarrhythmias.

The amount of energy an ICD is capable of delivering varies by manufacturer and model. In this context, it is important to recognize the distinction between stored energy and delivered energy so that unfair comparisons are not made. For instance, it is not a fair comparison to say that an ICD with 36 J of *stored energy* is equivalent to an ICD with 36 J of *delivered energy*. In the most simplistic terms, stored energy refers to the amount of energy that the capacitors can hold, while delivered energy refers to the amount of energy the capacitors release. Since no capacitor unloads all of its charge, stored energy is by definition always greater – sometimes a few joules larger, in fact. For clinical applications, the relevant information is the amount of energy a device can deliver.

Once the clinician has determined the proper energy value for therapy for the fib zone and tach zones, the device can be programmed. When an arrhythmia is detected, therapy will be delivered synchronously with the next non-sinus complex, that is, synchronously with the patient's next R-wave (see Fig. 8.1).

It is well known that many arrhythmic episodes self-terminate. So what happens if the device sees enough activity to detect an arrhythmia but as it prepares to deliver therapy (just a matter of seconds), sinus rhythm is restored? That depends on how the ICD is built. An ICD that is 'committed' will deliver therapy once an arrhythmia is detected, even if sinus rhythm resumes. The concept is that the system 'commits' to therapy at the detection point and delivers it – no matter what.

A 'noncommitted' device detects an arrhythmia, prepares for therapy, but will abort the shock if it detects that sinus rhythm is restored before therapy delivery. (Remember that what the device calls 'sinus rhythm' is based on programmable rate ranges and may not be the same thing as clinical sinus rhythm.) (See Fig. 8.2.)

When a shock is aborted, the capacitor has already started to store energy. In fact, it may be very near capacity. This shock now has nowhere to go. The device solves this problem by allowing the energy to dissipate gradually or 'bleed off.' (This may be available as a programmable feature called 'Dump Capacitors' which must be enabled.) When a charge bleeds off, the patient does not notice anything and there is no damage to the device.

One of the most important aspects of any ICD is charge time, that is, how much time is necessary after diagnosis for the device to charge to full capacity and administer life-saving therapy. Charge times can vary with the age of the device, battery status, state of the capacitors, and other factors. Theoretical charge times for devices are generally measured at the beginning of life and are usually around 10 seconds (see Fig. 8.3).

Engineers and clinicians have noticed that the type of waveform delivered can affect its therapeutic value. Very early in the history of ICDs, it was determined that biphasic waveforms were far more effective – even at identical settings – than monophasic

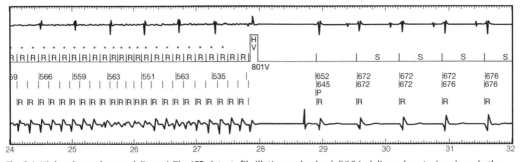

Fig. 8.1 High-voltage therapy delivered. The ICD detects fibrillation and a shock (HV) is delivered, restoring sinus rhythm.

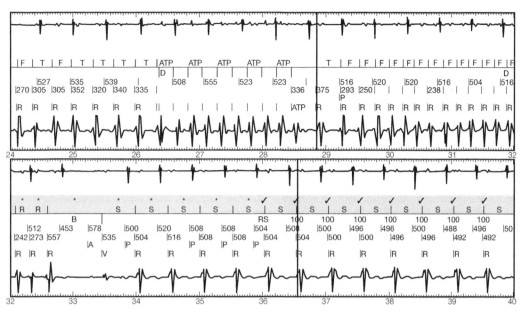

Fig. 8.2 Fib therapy aborted. This noncommitted device diagnoses an arrhythmia and delivers ATP, which accelerates the arrhythmia to ventricular fibrillation (VF). The device prepares to deliver therapy, but then sinus rhythm (as the device defines it) is restored (bottom strip). Since this is a noncommitted device, the shock is aborted. Had the ICD been a committed device, the therapy would have been delivered.

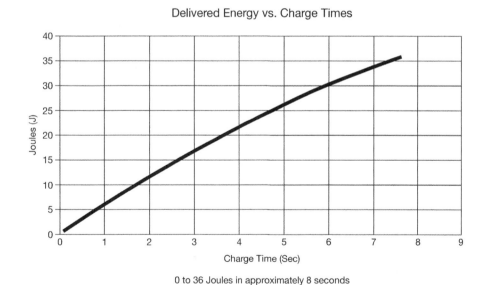

Fig. 8.3 Charge times. This graph shows the charge times for the Epic™+ ICD at its beginning of service. It charges to a maximum output of 30 joules in 7.2 seconds. Charge times will change over the life of the device and are fastest at the beginning of service.

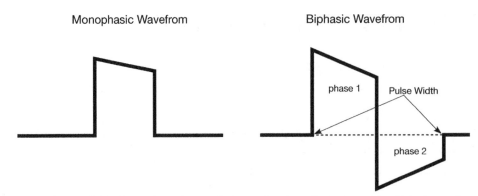

Fig. 8.4 Monophasic and biphasic waveforms. A monophasic waveform has a single phase while a biphasic waveform consists of an initial positive phase followed by a shorter negative phase.

waveforms at defibrillating the heart. A monophasic waveform is defined as a waveform that only goes in one direction with respect to the baseline. A biphasic waveform has two phases: a first positive phase (upward from baseline) followed by a second, shorter, negative phase (see Fig. 8.4).

Since a biphasic waveform can defibrillate the heart with less energy, it rapidly became the standard of care. However, no one knows exactly why the biphasic waveform works the way it does. While the exact cellular mechanisms remain unclear, it has been established that biphasic waveforms are more effective at defibrillating.

Are there other waveform morphologies that might also enhance defibrillation efficacy? One variable that is often discussed in this connection is called tilt. Tilt is defined as the percentage decrease in voltage at the capacitor measured from the lead-ing edge (start of first waveform) to the trailing edge of the pulse. Tilt is affected by the capacitance (that is, the state of the capacitor), the impedance of the lead system used with the ICD, and the duration of the therapy (see Fig. 8.5).

Clinical experience with varying tilts has given us information which seems counterintuitive. It would appear that a higher tilt – that is, a waveform that delivered more energy – would be more effective at defibrillating the heart. In fact, studies have shown that a tilt value in the range of 40–65% is actually more effective than higher tilt values of 80%.[3]

ICDs are designed to accommodate either a fixed tilt or a fixed pulse width when it comes to therapy output. In a fixed tilt system, the device has a firm and unchanging tilt for the waveform. The clinician programs the energy, but the tilt remains fixed. In order to deliver the right amount of energy at the

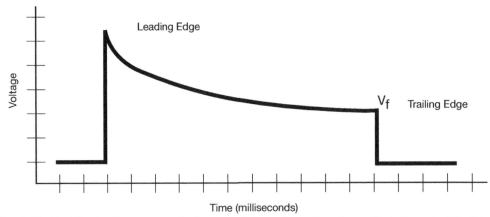

Fig. 8.5 Tilt: this defined as the percentage of voltage drop between the leading edge and the trailing edge (Vf) of the waveform.

fixed tilt, the device sometimes has to automatically adjust the pulse width (duration of output) to accommodate variations in impedance. When programming with a fixed tilt system, the device is programmed in joules (because the device adjusts everything to deliver the programmed amount of energy).

On the other hand, some ICDs are set up with a fixed pulse width. The clinician programs therapy by selecting voltage and pulse width values. The tilt is then adjusted to accommodate those settings. With fixed pulse width ICDs, the energy varies as lead impedance varies. Thus, fixed pulse width settings require the shock to be programmed in volts, since the device delivers the appropriate voltage, but pulse width (and thus total energy delivery) can vary.

The two systems: fixed tilt and fixed pulse width may be available as programmable options for the ICD. Further options may even allow clinicians to program fixed tilt or fixed pulse width independently for fib zones and tach zones. Likewise, monophasic and biphasic waveforms may also be programmable options.

Thus, clinicians programming shock therapy may have to select several values to define the shock. These items can usually be independently programmed by zone, that is, different values can be programmed for Tach A, Tach B, and fib.
- Monophasic or biphasic waveform.
- Programmable pulse width (in voltage) or programmable tilt (in joules).
- Shock parameters (in voltage or joules).

In addition to these parameters, it may be useful to reverse the polarity of a device. In a dual-coil ICD system, the electrical circuit is formed from the right ventricular (RV) coil at the distal tip of the RV lead to either the lead in the superior vena cava (SVC) and the ICD can or the ICD can alone. Programming the SVC coil 'on' or 'off' determines how the electrical circuit is formed. (With the SVC coil on, the circuit is from RV lead to SVC lead and can; with the SVC coil off, the circuit runs from RV lead to can.) Changing the polarity affects the shocking vectors, that is, the path the electrical energy takes through the heart during defibrillation. Changing shocking vectors may improve defibrillation efficacy in some patients. This is not a parameter that is frequently adjusted, but it can provide more flexibility for managing unusual cases.

Antitachycardia pacing (ATP)

ATP has long been recognized as a way to pace-terminate certain types of arrhythmias, but only certain rhythms (and certain patients) respond to it. Because ATP involves some special programming and is known to be ineffective (and sometimes even pro-arrhythmic) in some patients, many clinicians do not bother to program ATP options in ICDs. But ATP offers some powerful advantages and is usually worth considering:
- ATP is not painful; in fact, many patients do not even notice it.
- Although programming ATP requires some knowledge of programmed stimulation, setting it up can be fairly simple.
- Many hemodynamically stable VTs can be terminated without having to resort to painful shock therapy.
- ATP may reduce the drain on the battery by terminating some arrhythmias without shocks.

The ideal candidate for ATP is an asymptomatic patient who is susceptible to reentrant monomorphic VT but remains hemodynamically stable. In other words, you do not want to program ATP when the patient is unstable, hemodynamically compromised, or suffering. However, many patients do develop such VTs and ATP can be an effective, painless, almost 'invisible' way of managing them.

ATP only works on monomorphic VT involving a reentry circuit. This arrhythmia requires a bypass tract or closed loop, which must have unidirectional block plus a fast side and a slow side. This constellation of conditions results in a reentry circuit. Electricity traveling into the closed loop makes its way down the fast side of the loop first. This electricity is already out of the loop as electricity travels the slower leg. When the electricity reaches the lowermost portion of the loop, some of it will travel downward and out, but some of that slower energy will get deflected and travel back up the fast side and then back down the fast leg again. This cycle continues, getting faster and faster. (See Fig. 8.6.)

The theory behind ATP is the same as for programmed stimulation used in the EP lab: one or several carefully timed low-voltage pacing impulses are delivered to the heart at a rate faster than the tachycardia in order to break the 'vicious cycle' of the reentry loop and terminate the arrhythmia.

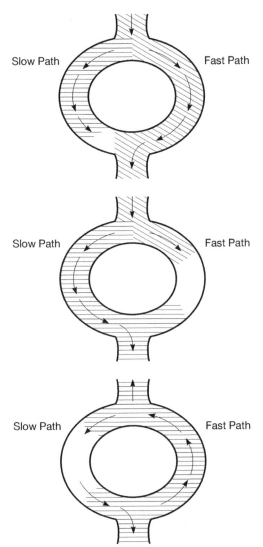

Fig. 8.6 Reentrant VT. A reentrant circuit requires a closed loop with a fast side and a slow side. Electricity entering the loop splits, with some electricity traveling down the fast path and some down the slow path. The electricity is already through the fast path and tissue on that side of the circuit starts to repolarize so that it is no longer refractory at about the same time that the electricity reaches the lowest portion of the slow path. Now, instead of traveling down and out of the loop, some of that electricity is able to split off and travel back up the fast path. This creates a circular pathway with electricity traveling faster and faster through the loop. The electrical energy 'reenters' the fast path (reentry tachycardia) and travels backward. The difference in electrical conduction properties in the loop keep the energy circling around the bypass tract, faster and faster.

While just one single properly timed output pulse can effectively terminate a tachycardia, most ATP sequences involve multiple outputs in a precisely timed pattern.

There are a few drawbacks to ATP therapy that must be considered as well. ATP takes some time, because not only does the ICD have to detect the arrhythmia, the programmed stimulation sequence can take several moments. Many ATP sequences involve multiple attempts to terminate a VT, which can mean that the entire ATP therapy takes several minutes. This is not appropriate if the patient is hemodynamically compromised or experiencing symptoms. While ATP is effective at terminating VT, it can sometimes accelerate the rhythm rather than interrupt it. If this acceleration is great and if the patient might be susceptible to having VF develop from VT, this involves considerable risk that the ATP will provoke a more severe arrhythmia rather than terminate a relatively benign one. For these reasons, ATP is generally preferred for patients who experience stable, asymptomatic VTs at rates below 200 bpm.

ATP programming involves setting up a pattern of stimulation outputs to be used when the device detects a VT. The main drawback to ATP is that it may accelerate a VT into VF. For that reason, ATP should be used with care, typically in patients who have tachyarrhythmias that are known to respond to ATP.

To understand how to program ATP, it is useful to learn the lingo, which differs from normal pacing terminology (see Table 8.1).

The decision as to how to program ATP for an individual patient should be based on the clinician's experience both with programmed stimulation and the particular patient. The clinician would first set up the train: this might consist of an individual extrastimulus or a rapid sequence of stimuli (burst). The burst cycle length (BCL) determines the speed of the impulse. Since ATP is based on the notion that pacing at a rate above the tachycardia rate terminates the VT, the BCL should be greater than the VT. Thus, if the ICD has a Tach A range for VTs of 150–200 bpm, the BCL for ATP therapy in that zone should be greater than 200 bpm, which works out to a cycle length of 300 ms or below. This involves programming the BCL to a fixed value.

Many devices allow the BCL to be dynamically based on the rate of the intrinsic VT and pro-

Table 8.1 ATP terms

ATP term	Meaning
Extrastimulus	A single, precisely timed pacing output pulse
Burst	1. A sequence of precisely timed output pulses
	2. A pattern of programmed stimulation that may include several bursts or extrastimuli
Train	This is the same as no. 2 of burst (see above)
Burst cycle length (BCL)	The programmable parameter that controls the speed of the ATP output pulses
Ramp pacing	Increasing the pacing rate (that is, decreasing the cycle length) within one individual burst
Scanning	Changing the cycle length (that is, increasing or decreasing the rate) from one burst to the next burst
Attempt	The use of a burst or train to terminate a VT
Readapt	A programmable parameter that allows a burst to change automatically as the VT cycle length changes

grammed as an adaptive or percentage value. In this case, the cycle length is automatically adjusted to a percentage value of the current VT cycle length. For instance, the BCL can be programmed to the adaptive setting of 85%, which means that each burst will be automatically adjusted by the device so that it is 85% of the tachycardia cycle. When adaptive BCL is used, the device is said to readapt, that is, adjust the cycle length (see Fig. 8.7).

When programming a burst, that is, a series of rapid stimulating outputs, the clinician will also be asked to program the number of stimuli in that burst. In theory, only one extrastimulus is needed to terminate a VT, but the programmable range for number of stimuli ranges from 2 to 20 with 6 a good default value.

Setting up a BCL and a number of stimuli defines one individual burst. Sometimes a clinician will set up a train that involves multiple bursts (often programmable from 1 to 15). For example, the ICD can be set up to deliver a rapid series of six output pulses, then pause, and then deliver another six, and so on until it completes a dozen bursts. When ATP is programmed that way, the burst is a sequence of six pulses and the train is the series of a dozen bursts.

Ramping allows output pulses within a burst to be decreased by a programmable amount from one pulse to the next (see Fig. 8.8). Sometimes called 'autodecrementing,' each output is shorter (by the programmed step value) than the one preceding it within that burst.

Scanning allows a burst to be delivered and if the VT persists, the next burst will be delivered at a faster rate (see Fig. 8.9).

Ramp pacing and scanning can be programmed together, so that the ATP will pace more and more

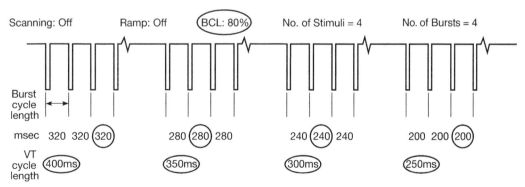

Fig. 8.7 Adaptive BCL. Readapted ATP allows the burst cycle length (BCL) to automatically adjust to a percentage value of the tachycardia cycle length. In the first sequence, the VT cycle length is 400 ms and the programmed 80% BCL results in a burst cycle length of 320 ms (0.80 × 400). As the VT cycle length changes, so does the BCL. In the last sequence in the illustration, the VT cycle length is just 250 ms and the BCL is 200 ms (0.80 × 250).

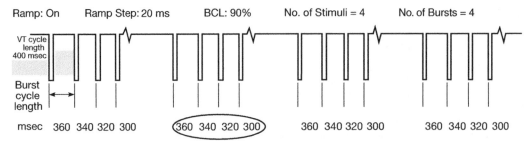

Fig. 8.8 ATP ramping. In this example, four bursts are programmed with four output pulses to a burst. The burst cycle length is programmed to 90%. Ramp is on with a ramp step value of 20 ms. This means that each successive pulse in an individual burst is 20 ms shorter than the one preceding it. Ramping only affects outputs *within a burst*.

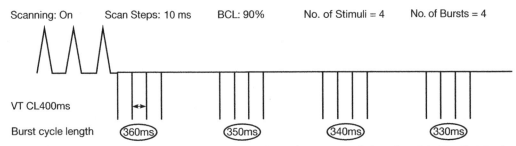

Fig. 8.9 ATP scanning. In this example, scanning is programmed on with a scan step of 10 ms. The BCL is 90%. The VT cycle length is 400 ms, so the BCL is 360 ms (0.90 × 400). Each burst is 10 ms (the scan step) shorter than the burst preceding it. Scanning decreases from burst to burst.

rapidly, both within an individual burst and from one burst to the next, if the VT does not terminate (see Fig. 8.10).

Another useful ATP parameter involves adding stimuli per burst if a burst is unsuccessful (see Fig. 8.11). This is programmable and adds one pulse per burst after every unsuccessful burst, up to a maximum value (typically 20 pulses). These added pulses may increase the effectiveness of ATP. If ramping is programmed, the additional pulse will come in at the faster rate.

Redetection is employed, similar to that used for high-energy therapy, to ascertain the restoration of sinus rhythm. If sinus rhythm is not redetected, ATP continues according to the values to which it was programmed. When sinus rhythm is restored, ATP ceases.

Conclusion

An advanced, full-featured ICD allows the device to define and diagnose up to four different types of rhythms (sinus, slow VT, fast VT, fib). Just as this level of categorization is not necessary or even appropriate for some patients, not all patients will need ATP or cardioversion. However, for patients with multiple rhythm disorders, the ability to categorize and differentially treat these arrhythmias is a major advancement in ICD therapy. All ICDs require a fib zone with high-energy therapy delivery. For many patients, that may be all that is ever required. Yet for patients with slow VTs, ATP may be a painless solution. For those with hemodynamically stable fast VTs, cardioversion (lower-energy shocks) may be a therapeutic option. These refinements may make ICD therapy a bit more complicated at the outset, but they offer flexibility to meet the current and often changing needs of the patients who get these devices.

References

1 Shukla HH, Flaker GC, Jayam V, Roberts D. High defibrillation thresholds in transvenous biphasic implantable defibrillators: clinical predictors and prognostic implications. *Pacing Clin Electrophysiol* 2003; **26**: 44–8.

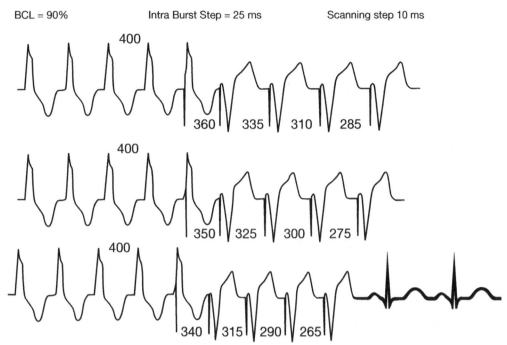

BCL = 90%   Intra Burst Step = 25 ms   Scanning step 10 ms

Fig. 8.10 ATP with ramping and scanning. This ATP sequence both ramps (decreases cycle length from output to output within a burst) and scans (decreases the cycle length from burst to burst). The VT cycle length is 400 ms and the BCL is adapted at 90%, resulting in an initial output of 360 ms (0.90 × 400). The intraburst step is 25 ms, so each output is 25 ms shorter than the one preceding it (360, 335, 310, 285). A burst is four outputs. In this example, the next burst follows the same pattern, but commences with a 10 ms shortening (scanning step of 10 ms). Thus, the next burst starts at 350 ms and the one after that starts at 340 ms. Ramping and scanning together allow for particularly aggressive ATP therapy.

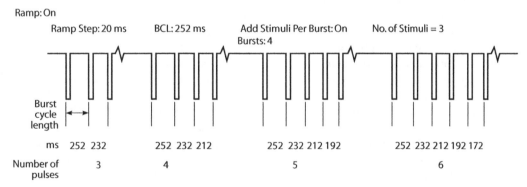

Ramp: On

Ramp Step: 20 ms   BCL: 252 ms   Add Stimuli Per Burst: On   No. of Stimuli = 3
                                                 Bursts: 4

Burst cycle length

ms   252 232   252 232 212   252 232 212 192   252 232 212 192 172

Number of pulses   3   4   5   6

Fig. 8.11 ATP with added stimuli. The feature 'Add stimuli per burst' is used to add one output pulse per burst after every unsuccessful burst. Since ramp is on, the additional outputs come in at the higher, ramped rate.

2   Qi X, Dorian P. Antiarrhythmic drugs and ventricular defibrillation energy requirements. *Chin Med J* 1999; **112**: 1147–52.

3   Yamanouchi Y, Brewer JE, Donohoo AM *et al.* External exponential biphasic versus monophasic shock waveform: efficacy in ventricular fibrillation of longer duration. Pacing Clin Electrophysiol 1999; **22**: 1481–7.

The nuts and bolts of arrhythmia therapy

- ICDs with tiered therapy offer antitachycardia pacing (ATP), cardioversion for ventricular tachycardia (VT), and defibrillation for ventricular fibrillation (VF), which can be programmed to meet the specific needs of the individual patient.
- In an ICD, cardioversion refers to therapy delivery for VT and is typically 2–15 joules.
- Joule is a unit of energy and volt is a unit for electromotive force. Both are sometimes used to define ICD output, with joule the more common term.
- ICDs can deliver high-energy (or high-voltage) outputs even though they have small (3.2 volt) batteries because capacitors are able to store a charge and then release it all at once.
- Capacitors can become deformed with lack of use and periodically require maintenance in the form of reformation. Reforming the capacitors is often automatic and involves fully charging the capacitors and then allowing the charge to dissipate harmlessly.
- The defibrillation threshold (DFT) is the amount of energy required to reliably defibrillate the heart during a life-threatening arrhythmia. DFT testing may be done at implant (often it is not). DFTs can change over time, with drugs, and with disease progression.
- Stored energy refers to how much energy can be stored in the device's capacitor, while delivered energy refers to how much energy is actually sent to the heart. Since capacitors cannot completely discharge, stored energy is always more than delivered energy, sometimes even several joules more.
- A noncommitted device will abort therapy if sinus rhythm (as the ICD defines it) is detected after an arrhythmia has been detected but before therapy is delivered. A committed device will not abort therapy in the same scenario. When therapy is aborted, the charge is dissipated gradually (or 'bled off') and is not felt by the patient.
- Charge time refers to the amount of time in seconds it takes for a device to fully charge and deliver therapy after an arrhythmia is detected. Charge times can be affected by many factors including the age of the device, battery status, and the condition of the capacitors. Most stated charge times refer to new devices (beginning of battery life).
- The morphology of the output waveform can be described as monophasic (one phase, positive with respect to the baseline) or biphasic (two phases, with a longer positive phase followed by a shorter negative phase). Biphasic waveforms are more effective at defibrillating the heart, but the reasons for this are unclear.
- Tilt refers to the percentage the voltage value decreases from the start of a defibrillation output (leading edge of the waveform) to the end of it (trailing edge of the waveform). Tilt can be a fixed value, in which the device alters other parameter values to maintain a constant tilt value, or it can be programmable. Studies show that a tilt value of 40–65% is most efficacious for defibrillation.
- Some devices allow for a fixed pulse width, in which case the device adjusts tilt and energy to maintain a constant pulse width value during a defibrillation output.
- Programmable polarity, also called programmable shocking vectors, allows the clinician to program the defibrillation energy circuit. It can either be the right ventricular (RV) lead to the SVC lead and can or it can be the RV lead to the can. Programmable shocking vectors can improve defibrillation efficacy in some patients.
- Antitachycardia pacing (ATP) is a form of programmed stimulation that can be effective in some patients to terminate an asymptomatic,

Continued.

Continued.

hemodynamically stable VT, particularly one that is under 200 bpm.

- ATP involves programming attempts or trains that are made of up of extrastimuli (individual outputs) or bursts (a series of outputs). These outputs can be programmed to a fixed burst cycle length (say 300 ms) or an adaptive value (for example, 85% of the patient's current tachycardia cycle length). When bursts are adaptive, the process by which the cycle length is determined is sometimes called readaptation.

- Several ATP sequences may be required to terminate a VT. Ramping allows the burst cycles to be decrementing by a programmable amount (called the ramp step) and scanning allows burst cycle lengths to be changed from burst to burst. Ramps occur within bursts, scans occur burst to burst. ATP programming can use one or the other or both.

- In ATP programming, a clinician may find it useful to add a stimulus per burst in successive attempts to terminate a VT.

CHAPTER 9

SVT discrimination

Patients who get potentially life-saving high-voltage therapy from their ICD frequently report that therapy delivery is disturbing, unsettling, startling ... and painful. Therapy delivery can occur before the patient notices any symptoms, and therapy can feel like getting kicked in the chest by a mule. Even patients who do not report such painful shocks still find therapy delivery alarming, for it brings them uncomfortably close to the notion of their own mortality and dependence on a device. For these reasons and for the sake of battery longevity, it is important that ICDs shock the patient only when necessary.

Yet in the quest to make ICDs as responsive as possible to life-threatening arrhythmias, many clinicians can program settings which also make the device responsive to arrhythmic activity that the ICD was not designed to treat. Such shocks are called inappropriate, and they can tax the patient, drain the device battery, and place an unnecessary burden on the local physicians, clinics, and hospitals that may be visited by these patients for treatment.

ICDs are designed to treat life-threatening ventricular tachyarrhythmias, which, by definition, are rhythm disorders that originate in the ventricles. However, many rhythm disorders originate above the ventricles. Supraventricular tachycardia (SVT) refers to a broad class of tachyarrhythmias which are known to start in the atria or AV node. Since SVTs often conduct down to the ventricles and provoke a rapid ventricular response, the ICD may detect a rapid ventricular rate and 'mistake' it for a tachycardia that is ventricular in origin.

SVTs include such common rhythm disorders as atrial fibrillation (AF), atrial flutter, and atrial tachycardia. It is no rarity for an ICD patient to have multiple rhythm disorders, and one study estimated that about 50% of all current ICD patients would develop AF over the course of their lifetime.[1] It is

no wonder that one study found a 14% incidence of inappropriate therapy delivery in ICD patients[2] (earlier papers reported even higher rates for older devices[3]), which bears out what many clinicians have observed in clinical practice. The documented presence of atrial tachyarrhythmias prior to ICD implantation has been identified as a risk factor for inappropriate ICD therapy, but inappropriate therapy delivery can potentially affect any ICD patient.[4]

The ICD constantly monitors the patient's ventricular rate. When a certain number of intervals at the cut-off rate (or above) are counted, the ICD 'detects' the arrhythmia. At this point (and it takes just moments), the ICD then 'diagnoses' the arrhythmia by categorizing it as Tach A, Tach B or fib. Once the diagnosis is made, the ICD prepares to deliver therapy. The entire process may take fewer than 10 seconds.

The problem arises in that the ICD can only monitor the ventricular rate. It has no way of knowing whether a 200 bpm ventricular rate is the result of rapid response to AF or whether it is ventricular tachycardia (VT). Likewise, a patient with a 200 bpm ventricular rate may be experiencing an exercise-induced sinus tachycardia. Therapy delivery to such patients is inappropriate.

In order to develop an ICD that had good sensitivity (that is, identified VT and VF reliably) as well as good specificity (that is, could tell the difference between SVT and VT/VF), engineers have developed special algorithms known broadly as SVT discriminators to be sure that an ICD detected and treated every VT/VF but did not deliver therapy to SVT. SVT discriminators are algorithms available in Tach A and Tach B zones. (SVT discriminators cannot be used in the fib zone.)

SVT discrimination settings are programmable, and the entire SVT discrimination function can be programmed off or, in some devices, to a passive setting which allows clinicians to see how the SVT discriminators would have classified a rhythm disorder (but does not allow the SVT discrimination to impact diagnosis and therapy). The passive function can be particularly useful when assessing the value of new or different SVT discriminators.

The theory behind SVT discrimination is the same clinical judgment that doctors and nurses use every day when assessing a patient's ECG or intracardiac electrogram. For example, when a patient has a rapid ventricular rate, most clinicians would examine that patient's atrial rate. Is there some form of atrial tachyarrhythmia? Clinicians would also check as to whether the rhythm disorder started gradually or abruptly. A ventricular arrhythmia often starts abruptly. A discerning clinician would examine the ventricular rate for regularity, stability, and the morphology of the QRS complex. If the QRS complex looks normal, then there is a good chance that the rhythm is conducted. But if the QRS is distorted, then it suggests that there is a different site of origin for the arrhythmia. ICDs use these very same techniques in the form of algorithms incorporated in the device.

Rate Branch

Available in dual-chamber ICDs only, Rate Branch is a fairly straightforward algorithm that has considerable power to discriminate SVTs from VTs (see Fig. 9.1). In old-fashioned diagnosis of an arrhythmia with a known rapid ventricular rate, most clinicians would immediately look at the atrial rate. If the ventricular rate is the result of rapid response

to an atrial tachyarrhythmia, then the atrial rate should be faster than the ventricular rate. By the same token, a tachycardia originating in the ventricles (VT) would not involve the atria, which would be beating at a normal rate.

The ICD determines the patient's ventricular rate and the patient's simultaneous atrial rate. If the ventricular rate is less than the atrial rate (V < A), then the device diagnoses this as atrial flutter or AF. This is an SVT and the ICD would automatically inhibit therapy.

On the other hand, if V > A, that is, the ventricular rate was more rapid than the atrial rate, the ICD would categorize this as VT and advance to deliver therapy.

In some cases, V = A, that is, there is 1:1 synchrony between atria and ventricles. In such cases, the ICD determines that this is either a sinus tachycardia or a rapid ventricular response to an atrial tachycardia. In either case, therapy is withheld (see Fig. 9.2).

In actual clinical practice, rhythm disorders can be deceptive. For example, what about a patient who has underlying chronic atrial fibrillation (AF) and develops a slow VT? The Rate Branch algorithm would regard that as an SVT because the atrial rate surpasses the ventricular rate. For that reason, another SVT discriminator is available which helps to sort out rapid ventricular rates caused specifically by AF.

Interval Stability

AF is a very rapid, erratic rhythm which conducts inconsistently through the AV node. The rapid ventricular response associated with AF is characterized

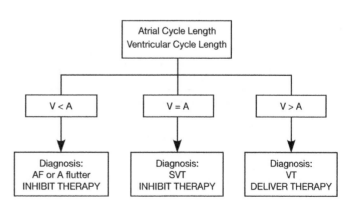

Fig. 9.1 Rate discrimination. Rate branch compares the atrial and ventricular rates to reach its diagnosis, much as a clinician would do looking at an ECG. If V < A (that is, the ventricular rate is slower than the atrial rate), then the ICD diagnoses a supraventricular tachycardia. If V = A (that is, the ventricular rate is the same as the atrial rate), then the ICD diagnoses a supraventricular tachycardia. In both such cases, the ICD will inhibit therapy delivery. However, if V > A (the ventricular rate is faster than the atrial rate), the ICD diagnoses VT and will deliver the programmed therapy.

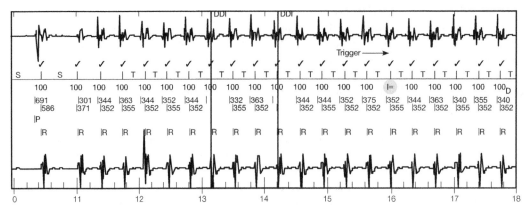

Fig. 9.2 Therapy inhibited by rate branch. In this tracing, a tachycardia was detected (notice the row of Ts in the upper half of the strip). Rate Branch found that there was one-to-one correspondence in atrial and ventricular rates (V = A). This resulted in inhibition of therapy, shown on the strip as I= (therapy was inhibited because V = A).

by an irregular ventricular rhythm. On the other hand, a tachycardia originating in the ventricles usually has a more regular, albeit rapid rhythm. Thus, Interval Stability is a special SVT discriminator which assesses the stability of the ventricular rate. Interval stability in the form of regular R–R intervals is diagnosed as a VT (therapy is delivered), while instability in the R–R intervals is diagnosed as AF with rapid ventricular response, inhibiting therapy.

The default setting for interval stability may be a delta or variance of 80 ms. If the R–R interval changes by more than 80 ms over a programmed number of intervals, the rhythm is determined to be irregular. This leads to a diagnosis of AF with rapid ventricular response; no therapy is initiated.

On the other hand, if the R–R interval does not vary by the programmed delta value over the programmed number of intervals, the rhythm is diagnosed as VT and therapy is delivered.

For dual-chamber ICDs, Rate Branch can be combined with Interval Stability to enhance SVT discrimination. In single-chamber ICDs, Interval Stability can be used alone as an SVT discriminator. (See Fig. 9.3.)

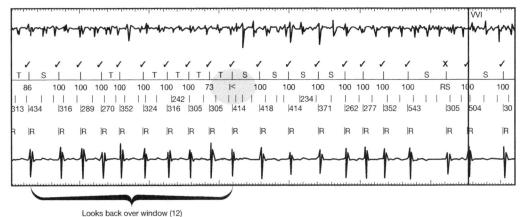

Looks back over window (12)
Compares 2nd shortest with 2nd longest
interval and calculates a difference or **DELTA**

Fig. 9.3 Therapy inhibited using interval stability. Here, the ICD detects a tachycardia (Ts) but determines that the interval stability varies by more than the programmed delta over the past 12 intervals. This means that the VT is irregular which, in turn, means that the tachyarrhythmia is actually an SVT (rapid ventricular response to AF). Therapy is inhibited.

Sudden Onset

Sinus tachycardia is the result of an atrial tachycardia in a heart with a relatively intact conduction system. Sometimes sinus tachycardia is the appropriate result of exertion or stress, while other times it is a relatively 'normal' ventricular response to an abnormal atrial tachyarrhythmia (not AF). Patients who get sinus tachycardia present a special dilemma for the ICD's discrimination algorithms. Patients who get both dangerous forms of VT and appropriate sinus tachycardia may have sinus tachycardia at rates that exceed the VT rates. Diagnosing rhythm disorders that fall in this 'overlap' area of appropriate sinus tachycardia and potentially dangerous (and treatable) VT requires a special discrimination algorithm known as Sudden Onset.

Sinus tachycardia is characterized by a gradual onset, often brought about by physiological demand. On the other hand, VT tends to start abruptly. Thus, just as a clinician might scan an ECG to see if a rapid ventricular rate came on suddenly or built up gradually, the Sudden Onset algorithm looks at the change (delta) in interval measurement from nontachycardia to a binned tachycardia interval. For instance, if the sudden onset delta was programmed to a typical value of 100 ms, the SVT discriminator would see if the change (from nontachycardia to tachycardia intervals) is less than or greater than the programmable delta. If the actual change is greater than the programmed delta (in this case, > 100 ms) then the device diagnoses the arrhythmia as VT and delivers therapy. On the other hand, if the actual change is less than the programmed delta (again, using our example < 100 ms), then the device diagnoses this rhythm disorder as an SVT and withholds therapy (see Fig. 9.4).

Sudden Onset may be used together with AV Rate Branch (in dual-chamber devices) or alone (in single-chamber systems).

Morphology Discrimination

Just as an experienced clinician would examine the morphology (shape) of QRS complexes on an ECG to help gain insight into the origin of an arrhythmia, the Morphology Discrimination (MD) algorithm allows that same sort of morphology comparison to occur – except it is done automatically as an SVT discrimination algorithm. It has long been known that the morphology of the QRS complex on an ECG varies in shape depending on where the beat originates. In an SVT, the initial impulse originates in the atria (or at least above the ventricles) and travels through the His–Purkinje network to the ventricles. This produces a characteristic waveform that varies somewhat between patients but is relatively consistent within a single patient.

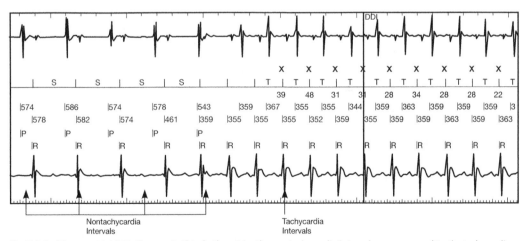

Fig. 9.4 Sudden onset inhibits therapy. In this rhythm strip, the nontachycardia intervals are compared to the tachycardia interval and the difference or change (delta) is compared to a programmable delta value. If the difference exceeds the programmed delta, then the arrhythmia is diagnosed as VT and therapy is delivered. If the difference is less than the programmed delta, then the arrhythmia is diagnosed as an SVT and therapy is inhibited.

VT, on the other hand, originates in the ventricles, does not involve His–Purkinje conduction, and results in a different QRS morphology on the ECG. Thus, by storing a QRS known to be caused by a beat originating in the atrium, subsequent QRS complexes could be compared and 'matched' (or not matched) to that QRS morphology. QRS complexes of similar shape would be presumed to be ventricular beats of atrial origin (and when the ventricular rate is rapid, this would indicate an SVT). By contrast, QRS complexes of significantly different morphology would be presumed to be ventricular in origin and any rapid ventricular rate would be the result of a VT (see Fig. 9.5).

Since there is considerable patient-to-patient variation in QRS morphology, the Morphology Discrimination requires the clinician to first establish a template for a sinus QRS. This is done when the algorithm is first activated at a programming session. Since heart patients may have conditions which change over time and affect the QRS shape, the template can be updated manually at subsequent follow-ups or even automatically. This template becomes the standard against which QRS complexes are evaluated.

When an arrhythmia interval is first detected, the process of morphology 'scoring' begins. Scoring continues until an arrhythmia is diagnosed. The ICD compares the arrhythmic QRS waveforms to the stored sinus template. If a match is made (and the nominal settings for match are 60%, but this value can be adjusted), then the ICD diagnoses the arrhythmia to be sinus in origin, that is, an SVT and therefore inhibits therapy. The match has to meet or exceed the programmed percentage criteria for a programmable number of intervals (for example, five out of eight intervals).

On the other hand, if a non-match is determined over a period of intervals, the arrhythmia is diagnosed as VT. These results are annotated on the stored electrogram. (See Fig. 9.6.)

Morphology Discrimination can be used in single- or dual-chamber ICD systems and can be used in conjunction or without other SVT discriminators. (See Fig. 9.7.)

Programming SVT discriminators

While SVT discriminators are individually fairly easy to understand, programming an ICD for SVT discrimination requires an appreciation of how all of these criteria could potentially interact. If only one discriminator is used, it is easy. But if several are used – in particular with AV Rate Branch – then a decision has to be made as to which criterion or criteria determine the diagnosis. For example, if Rate Branch and Morphology Discrimination and Sudden Onset are all programmed on, is the arrhythmia diagnosed if Rate Branch determines it is VT but Morphology Discrimination does not? And what if Rate Branch and Morphology Discrimination both indicate a VT … must Sudden Onset also agree or can therapy be delivered without it? (See Fig. 9.8.)

Using several SVT discriminators helps to assure the most reliable arrhythmia diagnosis. When possible, it is recommended that clinicians take advantage of these algorithms, except in cases when they might possibly provide confounding or misleading information. Some devices offer a special safety feature called Maximum Time to Diagnosis or Maximum

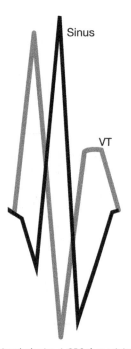

Fig. 9.5 QRS Morphologies. A QRS that originates from the sinus is typically narrower and 'sharper' than a QRS that originates from a ventricular source. In this example, the normally conducted QRS complex is darker, while the QRS of a ventricular tachyarrhythmia appears lighter.

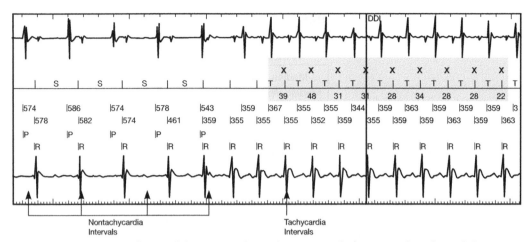

Fig. 9.6 MD inhibits therapy. This stored electrogram indicates that once an arrhythmia interval was detected, the Morphology Discrimination went into action. The T annotation indicates a tachycardia interval. The numbers below (39, 48, 31) indicate the percentage match compare to the stored waveform. The X above indicates an interval in which the match criterion was not met. In this case, the match had to be 60% in five out of eight tachycardia intervals. The match was not made, so the ICD diagnosed this arrhythmia as a VT and would prepare for therapy.

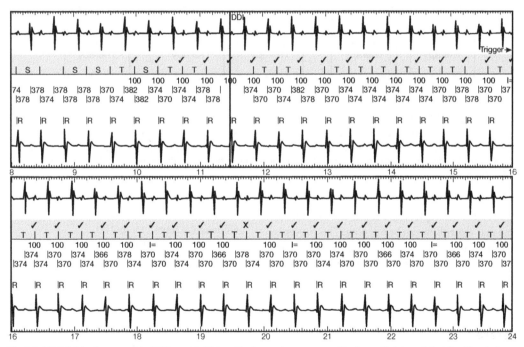

Fig. 9.7 MD inhibits therapy with 100% match. This patient experiences a run of tachycardia intervals but the Morphology Discrimination match (note the series of 100 annotations for 100% match) allows the device to diagnose an SVT and withhold therapy. Without SVT discrimination, this patient would likely have been subjected to a series of painful and inappropriate shocks.

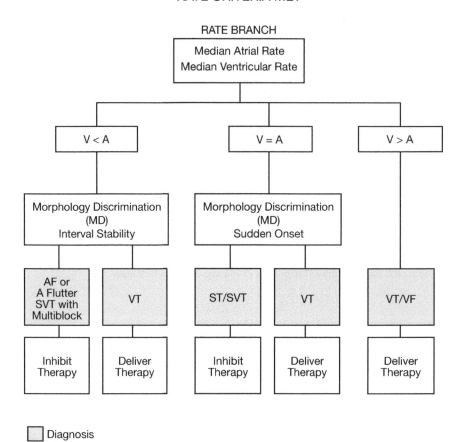

Fig. 9.8 SVT discrimination decision tree. This chart illustrates how the ICD uses algorithms to reach its diagnostic decisions. When high-rate ventricular activity is detected, the ICD first applies Rate Branch, then Morphology Discrimination and possibly other SVT discriminators to reach a decision as to the nature of the tachyarrhythmia and whether to deliver or inhibit therapy.

Time to Fib Therapy, which limits the amount of time that algorithms can be ongoing. This prevents SVT discriminators from withholding therapy over a prolonged period of time for a continuing rhythm disorder. This is covered in more detail in Chapter 12 (Special features).

References

1 Grimm W, Flores BF, Marchlinski FE. Electrocardiographically documented unnecessary spontaneous shocks in patients with implantable cardioverter defibrillators. *PACE* 1992; **15**: 1667–73.

2 Rinaldi CA, Simon RD, Baszko A *et al*. A 17-year experience of inappropriate shock therapy in patients with implantable cardioverter-defibrillators: are we getting any better? *Heart* 2004; **90**: 330–1.

3 Nunain SO, Roelke M, Trouton T *et al*. Limitations and late complications of third generation implantable cardioverter defibrillators. *Circulation* 1995; **91**: 2204–13.

4 Brugada J. Is inappropriate therapy a resolved issue with current implantable cardioverter defibrillators? *Am J Cardiol* 1999; **83**: 40D–44D.

The nuts and bolts of SVT discrimination

- Inappropriate therapy can distress the patient, drain the ICD battery, and place a burden on the clinicians who care for the patients. Minimizing or eliminating inappropriate therapy is very important for successful long-term ICD therapy.
- Inappropriate therapy is ICD therapy delivered in an attempt to terminate a rapid ventricular rate caused by a supraventricular tachycardia (SVT). An SVT is any tachyarrhythmia that originates above the ventricles.
- An ICD initially detects the ventricular rate interval. SVT discriminators come into play to help determine if the rapid ventricular rate is the result of an atrial tachyarrhythmia with rapid ventricular response or a ventricular tachycardia (VT).
- There are several available SVT discriminators which may be used individually or in combination. Available discriminators vary by device configuration (single-chamber versus dual-chamber) as well as by model and manufacturer.
- No SVT discriminators are available for the fib zone.
- The main SVT discriminators are Rate Branch (comparison of atrial and ventricular rates), Interval Stability, Sudden Onset, and Morphology Discrimination.
- Sensitivity means that an ICD can detect VT and VF; specificity means that it can distinguish between VT and SVT. 100% sensitivity is vital, but 100% specificity is not yet achievable.
- SVT discriminators use the same logic that a clinician would when studying an ECG with a rapid ventricular rate. They asses the atrial rate, the ventricular rate stability, and the QRS morphology.
- Rate Branch (available only in dual-chamber ICDs) compares the atrial to the ventricular rate. If A > V, then the arrhythmia is diagnosed as an SVT. If A = V, the arrhythmia is diagnosed as sinus tachycardia. In both cases, therapy is inhibited. On the other hand, if V > A, VT is diagnosed and therapy is delivered.
- Since patients can have AF simultaneously with a VT, Interval Stability compares R–R interval stability. If the R–R intervals are stable, the ICD diagnoses VT and proceeds to therapy. If the R–R intervals are unstable, the ICD assumes that AF is in progress, diagnoses SVT, and inhibits therapy.
- Sudden Onset compares nontachycardia intervals to tachycardia intervals and determines if the difference is greater than a programmable delta value (typically about 100 ms). If the difference exceeds the delta, the arrhythmia is determined to have started suddenly and is diagnosed as a VT. The ICD proceeds to therapy. On the other hand, if the difference does not exceed the delta, the arrhythmia is diagnosed as an SVT and therapy is withheld.
- Morphology Discrimination (MD) compares the patient's own sinus QRS complex to his or her QRS complexes during tachycardia and determines a match based on percentage (a 60% match is the nominal setting). If MD finds the proper degree of match in a programmable number of intervals (typically five out of eight), then the complexes match and the ICD diagnoses SVT and withholds therapy. On the other hand, if MD cannot match a sinus template to the current QRS complex in a programmable number of intervals, the ICD diagnoses VT and delivers therapy.
- When first programming Morphology Discrimination, the clinician obtains a sinus complex to use as a match. Since patients' conditions change over time, it is recommended to periodically update this template, either manually during subsequent programming sessions, or using an automatic update feature.
- While in theory it is a good idea to program the maximum amount of SVT discriminators, care must be taken to avoid programming discriminators in patients in whom confounding data might occur. Too many discriminators may cause the ICD to inhibit needed therapy.
- While SVT discrimination has not eliminated inappropriate therapy, when properly programmed, these algorithms can prevent unnecessary shocks in many patients.

CHAPTER 10

Bradycardia pacing

Defibrillators deliver therapy to the right ventricle. Common descriptions of ICDs such as 'single-chamber ICD' or 'dual-chamber rate-responsive ICD' or even the newer 'CRT-ICD' refer not to any refinement of the defibrillation capacity of the device, but to the low-voltage pacing therapy offered by the system. The first ICDs offered no bradycardia functionality, but gradually more and more pacemaker-type features were added. Today, it is possible to implant an ICD with all of the capabilities of a full-featured dual-chamber rate-responsive pacemaker. A new category of device incorporates cardiac resynchronization therapy devices (CRT devices which require a left ventricular lead) with an ICD. These devices are called CRT-D systems or sometimes CRT-ICDs.

Since it is not uncommon for some patients to have multiple rhythm disorders, some ICD patients also have standard bradycardia pacing indications. For these patients, the bradycardia features of an ICD should be programmed to provide them with the necessary rate support. Other ICD patients may not have a bradycardia indication, but may still benefit from post-shock pacing.

For the clinician following an ICD, it is important to program the pacing function properly. Unnecessary pacing has been shown to exacerbate heart failure, at least in some patients with compromised systolic function.[1] On the other hand, many patients with heart disease benefit from conventional pacing. The pacing prescription is adjusted by means of a variety of familiar pacing parameters.

Mode and timing parameters

The mode is a letter code system which describes where the pacing occurs (first letter), where sensing occurs (second letter), and what happens when an event is sensed (trigger, inhibit). A fourth letter may be used if rate-responsive settings and the sensor are active. Thus, DDDR pacing involves dual (both atrial and ventricle) pacing, dual sensing, a dual response (the device may trigger an output or inhibit an output when an intrinsic event is sensed), and has rate response. In VVI mode, the device paces and senses in the ventricle, inhibits in the presence of sensed activity, and has no rate response.

The most typical mode selections for ICD patients are DDDR, DDD, DDIR, DDI, VVIR, and VVI. So-called 'asynchronous pacing modes,' which do not sense but deliver output pulses regardless of the presence or absence of native activity, should only be used in ICD patients with extreme caution. Programming such a mode (DOO, VOO) may not be possible in an ICD, or may only be possible as a temporary setting or if the defibrillator function is turned off. Even in such limited applications, asynchronous pacing is not recommended in ICD patients because asynchronous pacing can result in the R-on-T phenomenon, in which a pacemaker output is delivered during the vulnerable portion of the T-wave, initiating a ventricular arrhythmia. Asynchronous pacing may also produce competitive pacing, that is, pacing which competes with intrinsic activity. If this occurs, the ICD might double-count the cardiac events (both sensed and paced) and deliver an inappropriate shock.

The base rate of the pacemaker refers to the rate at which the device will pace the heart in the absence of intrinsic activity. If the base rate is programmed to 70 ppm, the pacemaker will pace the heart whenever the intrinsic rate falls below 70 ppm. If the intrinsic rate is 70 ppm or greater, then the pacemaker output is inhibited. Pacemaker base rates are generally available in a range from about 40 ppm to 100 ppm, with 60 ppm nominal in most devices. Note that a higher base rate may require the pacemaker to pace more often, potentially using up battery reserves.

For patients who are not indicated for bradycardia pacing, programming a low base rate (for example, 40 ppm) assures that the device will be inhibited – that is, withhold delivery of an output pulse – most of the time, yet be available if the patient's heart rate ever drops to a very low level.

Rest rate is a relatively new pacemaker feature which allows the pacemaker to slow down during periods of sleep or profound inactivity. This allows the pacemaker to mimic the body's normal physiologic rate decrease during rest. Pacing at higher rates (say, 60 or 70 ppm) can be uncomfortable when a patient is trying to sleep. The rest rate may be programmed on or off, and when activated, may be set to a rate within a broad range (often about 35–95 ppm). Some devices rely on clock time, as programmed into the ICD, to determine when rest rate goes into effect and how long it lasts. Auto rest rate is a more advanced feature which uses the device's sensor to detect inactivity and then invokes the rest rate setting in 15–20 minutes after the patient has stopped activity. This frees the patient from having to sleep according to a prescribed bedtime and also allows the patient the benefits of rest rate during daytime naps or travel through different time zones.

Hysteresis allows the clinician to program a rate below the base rate which will inhibit the pacemaker. When hysteresis is activated, the pacemaker will pace at the programmed base rate (say 60 ppm). However, if hysteresis is programmed to 50 bpm, the pacemaker will remain inhibited as long as the patient's intrinsic rate is 50 bpm or higher. Hysteresis encourages the intrinsic activity to prevail, which is advantageous for most pacing patients. It also assures that pacing will occur if the native rate falls below a certain limit. Note that if a device had a base rate of 60 ppm and a hysteresis rate of 50 bpm, the device would not pace if the patient's rate was 55 bpm. However, if the patient's intrinsic rate was 49 bpm, the device would then commence pacing at the programmed base rate value of 60 ppm. For that reason, there should not be a vast gap between the programmed base rate and hysteresis rate. A special feature called 'search' allows the pacemaker to inhibit all pacing at regular intervals (typically every 5 minutes) for a brief period of time to allow intrinsic activity to break through and possibly inhibit the device. Hysteresis with search is one of the best tools to encourage a patient's intrinsic rhythm

to inhibit pacing, while still providing the benefits of potential pacing support if the rate drops below a certain level.

Rate-responsive ICDs usually require the clinician to activate a sensor function (typically On or Off) and then program some general rate-responsive settings. Rate-responsive pacing allows the pacemaker to increase the paced rate when the sensor determines that the patient is active. Likewise, when the patient is not active, the pacing rate goes back down to the programmed base rate. For active, younger, or fitter patients, rate-responsive settings help them maintain their vigorous lifestyle. Even patients who are not very active may still benefit from rate response.

When programming additional rate-responsive parameters, the main concern should be how aggressive the increase in rate should be to meet the patient's needs. The ICD may offer automated parameters such as Auto Slope and Auto Threshold which monitor stored data and adjust parameters based on the patient's previous activity. This requires minimal monitoring by the clinician (program on), yet fine-tunes rate response to meet the individual needs of the patient.

The AV delay is a routine pacemaker parameter, which requires careful adjustment in an ICD patient. This parameter allows the clinician to determine how much time must elapse between an atrial output and the next ventricular output (in the absence of intrinsic ventricular activity). Setting an AV delay affects the alert period of the device. A short AV delay creates a longer alert period, which allows the ICD to sense more intrinsic activity than a long AV delay would. For that reason, a short AV delay can enhance arrhythmia detection, while a long AV delay can limit arrhythmia detection. Most ICDs limit the programmable values for AV delay based on the programmed base rate. For example, if the base rate is set somewhere in the range of 45–85 ppm, then the maximum allowable AV delay is 350 ms. The programmer will not allow longer AV delays to be programmed.

The PV delay is a similar timing parameter, except that it sets the length of time between a sensed atrial event and the next ventricular output (in the absence of sensed ventricular activity). Typical values for the PV delay (sometimes called the sensed AV delay) range from about 25 to 325 ms.

An advanced parameter called Rate-Responsive AV/PV Delay may be available in some ICDs. This parameter is not a rate-responsive setting. It gets its name because it allows the AV/PV delay to vary in length in response to the patient's rate, thus mimicking the behavior of the healthy heart. If the patient's rate goes up, the AV/PV delay shortens automatically. This parameter is set by using values of high, medium, low and off, with the default setting of medium.

A very important pacing parameter for an ICD patient is the ventricular pace refractory period. This programmable setting determines an absolute refractory period – during which no activity is sensed – which is initiated by the delivery of a ventricular output pulse. This parameter is very important because it prevents the ICD from inappropriately sensing ventricular events and counting (or rather mis-counting) them. A wide range of ventricular refractory period settings may be available, typically in a range from about 135 to 470 ms with a nominal setting of around 250 ms.

Dual-chamber pacing allows the device to sense and pace the atrium and ventricle. Intrinsic atrial activity will cause the pacemaker to try to pace the ventricle to keep up and maintain 1:1 AV synchrony. When the patient's rate is relatively low, this 'atrial tracking,' as it is known, allows the pacemaker to mimic the healthy heart. For example, if a patient is walking up stairs and the sinus node starts to fire at around 90 or 100 bpm, the pacemaker will pace the ventricles in response to the atrium, delivering a ventricular output pulse in response to each sensed atrial event.

The problem with atrial tracking is atrial tachyarrhythmias. The Maximum Tracking Rate (MTR) is a programmable parameter which sets a 'speed limit' on how fast the ventricles can be paced in response to atrial activity. Thus, the MTR defines the highest rate at which the ventricles can be paced in response to atrial activity. In an ICD, it is also necessary to program a Tachy Detection Rate or other parameter which determines the rate at which therapy to terminate a VT is initiated. There has to be a buffer between the Tachy Detection Rate (when therapy is delivered) and the MTR, otherwise the system would pace the patient to the point of therapy delivery! Most ICDs do not allow the MTR rate to be programmed to a very high value.

While most programmers will not allow conflicting parameter values to be programmed, the calculation behind this is very simple. Convert both rates to intervals (ms settings) and make sure that the Tachy Detection Rate is at least 30 ms longer than the MTR. For example, if the Tachy Detection Rate was programmed to 150 bpm (400 ms), then the MTR should not be faster than 430 ms (140 bpm). An even bigger gap is probably better.

Pacing in the presence of atrial tachyarrhythmias was a challenge that was effectively countered many years ago in the pacemaker community by a special feature known as auto mode switch (AMS). If a dual-chamber pacemaker sensed very high-rate atrial activity (the value defining high-rate atrial activity could be programmed), it could effectively shut off the atrial channel until it determined that the atrial arrhythmia had terminated. This algorithm became known as mode switching because it automatically allowed a device to go from DDD to VVI pacing. (Some devices allow the clinician to program the modes that are involved in a mode switch, for example DDD to VVIR or VVI, while others provide automatic default values. In all cases, the atrial channel is turned off.) The device monitors the atrium and restores dual-chamber pacing as soon as normal atrial rates return.

The post-ventricular atrial refractory period (PVARP) is a dual-chamber pacemaker parameter which initiates a relative refractory period on the atrial channel after a sensed ventricular event or a ventricular output pulse (in DDI/R or DDD/R modes). During the PVARP, the device will not respond to any sensed atrial activity, but it will count atrial events. For example, if a P-wave occurs during the PVARP, it will not inhibit the atrial output pulse. However, that P-wave will be counted to update the atrial interval average counter of the Rate Branch discrimination algorithm. The PVARP is generally programmable over a wide range of settings, typically from 125 ms to 470 ms with a value of about 280 ms as a commonly used nominal setting.

Other advanced pacemaker parameters include PVC options and PMT options. The PVC Option allows the system to identify PVCs and automatically initiate a longer than normal PVARP. This decreases the possibility of a pacemaker-mediated tachycardia (PMT). PMT options (programmable to On, Off, or Passive) use a combination of retrograde conduction times and stability to identify PMT. (The clinician may also program the PMT detection rate, which determines how fast a PMT must occur before the algorithm is activated; the nominal setting for this is 90 ppm.) If a PMT is detected and the parameter 'A Pace on PMT' is programmed, the pulse generator withholds a ventricular output and delivers an atrial output pulse instead, 330 ms after the detected retrograde P-wave is sensed, in an effort to terminate the PMT. (See Table 10.1.)

Table 10.1 Characteristics of mode and timing parameters

Parameter	What it does	Typical values*	Comments
Mode	Programs how pacing and sensing are carried out	DDD, DDDR, VVI, VVIR, may be others	Avoid asynchronous modes (DOO, VOO)
Base rate	Determines how fast the pacemaker will pace in the absence of sensed activity	40–100 ppm; 60 ppm is a good default setting	A low base rate gives the patient's intrinsic rate more opportunity to prevail
Rest rate	Determines how low the base rate goes when the patient is resting	35–95 ppm, should be lower than the base rate	Auto Rest Rate uses a sensor to determine rest; some ICDs use clock time
Maximum tracking rate (MTR)	Determines the 'speed limit' or maximum ventricular pacing rate in response to tracked intrinsic atrial activity	90–150 ppm, nominal 110 ppm	Make sure this is lower by at least 30 ms (about 10 bpm) than the Tachy Detection Rate
2:1 Block rate	Not programmable, this is an automatic calculation on the programmer	Not programmable	Use to determine at what atrial rate 2:1 block will occur
Hysteresis	The pacemaker will not pace as long as the patient's intrinsic rate is at or above the programmed hysteresis rate	35–95 ppm, also Off	Should always be below the base rate. Allows patient's own intrinsic rate more opportunity to prevail
Hysteresis with search	Hysteresis which 'searches' regularly for intrinsic activity, giving maximum opportunity for intrinsic rate to break through	Search is on or off; typically searches every 5 minutes	Encourages patient's native rhythm to predominate
AV delay	Sets the timing cycle after an atrial output and before the next ventricular output pulse is delivered (in the absence of a sensed ventricular event)	35–350 ms, nominal is 170 ms	The AV delay affects the alert period of the ICD. The shorter the AV delay, the longer the alert period and consequently, the more opportunity the ICD has to detect arrhythmias
PV delay	Sets the timing cycle after an atrial sensed event and before the next ventricular output pulse is delivered (in the absence of a sensed ventricular event)	25–325 ms with a nominal setting of 150 ms	Always goes into effect when an atrial event is sensed
Rate-responsive AV/PV delay	Automatically shortens AV/PV delay when the patient's rate is higher than 90 ppm	High, medium, low, off	Has nothing to do with rate-responsive (accelerometer-related) settings
Post-ventricular atrial refractory period (PVARP)	An atrial relative refractory period that begins when the ICD senses an atrial event or PVC or ventricular output pulse (in some modes)	125–470 ms, nominal 280 ms	The ICD does not respond to atrial activity during PVARP, but still sees – and counts – atrial activity
Ventricular pace refractory	An absolute refractory period initiated by ventricular output	135–470 ms, nominal 250 ms	Prevents the inappropriate sensing of ventricular events; this period is absolute, so no events are counted or responded to

Continued p.74.

Table 10.1 *(Continued.)*

Parameter	What it does	Typical values*	Comments
Rate-responsive ventricular refractory period	Allows for ventricular refractory period to shorten automatically when the sensor-driven rates are above 90 ppm	High, medium, low, off	This has nothing to do with rate-responsive (accelerometer) settings
Shortest refractory period	Determines the shortest allowable ventricular refractory period value	125–470 ms, nominal 220 ms	Must be lower than the ventricular pace refractory value
Sensor	Activates accelerometer or other sensor for rate response	On, off	Useful in patients who may be active, fit, or are chronotropically incompetent
Auto mode switch	Temporarily turns off the atrial channel when atrial tachyarrhythmias are detected (thus, changes mode)	On, off, modes (DDIR to VVIR, and so on)	Useful when dual-chamber pacing is programmed in a patient with known atrial tachyarrhythmias
PVC options	Determines how the device responds when a PVC (as defined by ICD) occurs	Off or A Pace on PVC	Automatically extends PVARP in presence of PVC. Only available in DDD/R modes
PMT options	Determines how the device responds when a PMT is detected (PMT detection rate must also be programmed)	Off, passive, or A Pace on PMT	When PMT is determined and A Pace on PMT is programmed, the ICD will withhold a ventricular output in the presence of a PMT and deliver an atrial pulse 330 ms after the detected retrograde P-wave in an effort to terminate the PMT
PMT detection rate	Determines how the ICD defines a PMT	90–150 ppm, nominal 90 ppm	

*These settings describe rate ranges common in some ICDs. Actual rate ranges and nominal values will vary by manufacturer and even by model from a single manufacturer. For that reason, please use this chart only as a rough rule of thumb. Consult the device manual for specific information about a given ICD.

While pacemaker parameters may seem somewhat familiar to those used to dealing with low-voltage devices, there are some special considerations in how the pacing function of an ICD functions.

Episodal pacing

ICD patients typically experience tachycardia episodes, which may or may not culminate in therapy delivery. During a tachycardia episode, the amount of pacing should be reduced as much as possible to prevent acceleration of the arrhythmia or to avoid potential mis-counting. The device defines a tachycardia episode as starting with the binning of the very first interval of the tachycardia and counts the tachycardia episode as terminated when the device can detect a return to sinus rate (RS).

After three intervals are binned as tachycardia intervals, the fourth interval (if tachycardia) initiates episodal pacing. Unlike other device features, episodal pacing is not programmable and cannot be turned off. At the fourth tachycardia interval in the series, the pacemaker function of the ICD will:

- Switch the mode to DDI (dual-chamber systems) or VVI (single-chamber systems).
- Turn the sensor (if on) to Passive (thus disabling rate response).
- Disable ventricular safety standby (a cross-talk protection feature).
- Disable rate-responsive AV delay (an automatic shortening of the AV delay, which extends the alert period).
- Change the sensing threshold for bradycardia to the same as the sensing threshold for tachycardia.

These changes are all made in response to high-rate ventricular activity. Disabling rate response, disabling the automatic AV delay shortening in the presence of high rate, and switching to tachycardia sensing threshold settings all allow the device to focus on arrhythmia detection rather than pacing. Whether the device delivers therapy or the arrhythmia resolves spontaneously, episodal pacing ends when the device determines that normal sinus rhythm has resumed (see Fig. 10.1).

Post-shock pacing

Therapy delivery obviously affects cardiac tissue, and patients in the immediate post-therapy stage may respond more favorably to different pacing parameter settings than the values normally used in conventional pacing. Post-shock pacing (PSP) offers programmable values to the clinician which go into effect after high-voltage (defibrillation or cardioversion) or ATP (antitachycardia pacing) therapy has terminated an arrhythmia. (Note that PSP does not go into effect after the shock-on-T function, which is used during testing for arrhythmia induction.)

The clinician must first program a value for pause, which defines how many seconds must elapse after therapy and before the onset of PSP. Programmable values are usually between 1 and 7 seconds. It is generally recommended that some moments are allowed to elapse before commencing PSP, since immediate bradycardia pacing following a shock might be pro-arrhythmic. A few seconds can also give the traumatized cardiac tissue some time to recover.

Also programmable is the PSP duration, which defines how long PSP pacing parameters will be in effect. The programmable range is 30 seconds to 10 minutes. As a rule of thumb, the duration should be shorter in pacemaker-dependent patients (who need pacing support) and longer in those who can tolerate periods without pacing. In fact, when the clinician wants to inhibit competitive pacing (pacing on top of an intrinsic rhythm) or avoid higher sensor-driven rates, a longer duration is recommended.

For PSP, the clinician may program special mode, base rate, and output settings (pulse width and pulse amplitude). Available modes are non-rate-responsive. It is recommended that a lower than usual base rate be programmed, since faster base rates (even the conventional base rate) can accelerate the vulnerable cardiac tissue back into a tachyarrhythmia. Following a shock, the patient's capture threshold may be temporarily elevated. The best way to compensate for this higher than usual capture threshold is to increase output settings: program a higher than normal pulse amplitude or a longer than normal pulse width. (Increasing the pulse amplitude adds more energy than extending the pulse duration; it may be useful to do both.) The nominal output settings for PSP are high: 7.5 V (pulse amplitude) and 1.9 ms (pulse duration) and should not be decreased except with careful clinical consideration.

These are the general guidelines for PSP (see Fig. 10.2):
- Lower base rate than normal pacing.
- No rate response.
- Higher outputs than normal pacing.

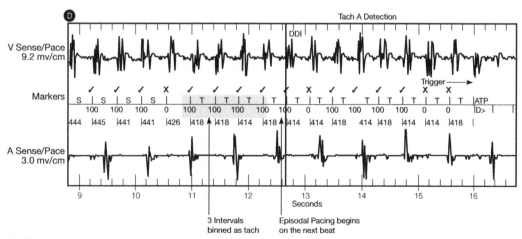

Fig. 10.1 Episodal pacing. Episodal pacing starts after four consecutive T events. Normal pacing will not resume until sinus rhythm is restored.

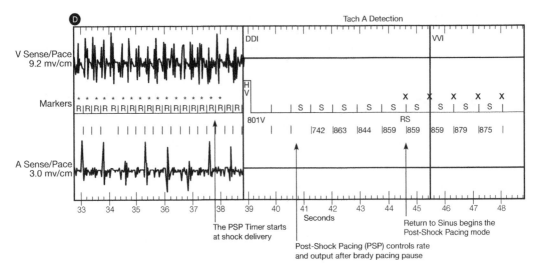

Fig. 10.2 Post-shock pacing. The ICD delivers a shock to terminate an episode of VF, which initiates the PSP timer. A pause of programmable duration ensues, followed by PSP at special PSP settings (slower base rate, higher outputs, no rate response). PSP is temporary and should be programmed to last only a short period of time (typically measured in seconds or a few minutes).

Special PSP parameters also go into effect after ATP or after a shock is aborted. In this case, the full range of PSP parameters do not go into effect. The only changes are:
- Rate-responsive AV delay is disabled.
- Sensor (accelerometer) is passive.

Reference

1   Wilkoff BL, Cook JR, Epstein AE *et al.* Dual-chamber pacing or ventricular backup pacing in patients with an implantable defibrillator: the Dual Chamber and VVI Implantable Defibrillator (DAVID) trial. *JAMA* 2002; **288**: 3115–23.

The nuts and bolts of bradycardia pacing

- Most ICDs offer full-featured pacemakers which allow a wide range of programmability to meet the needs of a broad base of patients. For patients with a bradycardia pacing indication, the ICD should be programmed to meet those needs.
- Some pacemaker parameters may affect how the ICD works and should be programmed judiciously. These include AV delay, rate-responsive settings, and the maximum tracking rate (which should always be lower than the tachy detection rate).
- If an ICD patient is not indicated for cardiac pacing, it is best to program the pacemaker to a very low base rate, which would keep the pacemaker inhibited most of the time.
- Episodal pacing occurs when the ICD detects a tachycardia. The purpose of episodal pacing is to minimize pacing during a potential tachyarrhythmic episode.
- Post-shock pacing (PSP) allows pacing at different parameters immediately following therapy, when cardiac tissue may be traumatized and vulnerable.
- In general PSP values are a low base rate and high output. The clinician must also program a pause (between therapy and onset of PSP) and duration of PSP. Pacemaker-dependent patients need a short period of PSP.

CHAPTER 11

Electrograms

The advent of implantable devices has given rise to the prevalence of the intracardiac electrogram, sometimes called an IEGM but more commonly known today as an electrogram or EGM. Unlike a surface ECG, which creates a tracing of the patient's cardiac rhythm based on electrical signals picked up from the surface of the skin, an intracardiac electrogram relies on the sensing capabilities of the lead electrodes located within the heart itself. An electrogram is an 'inside look' at what is going on in the heart. In the EGM, the lead reports what it 'sees' going on in the heart. Thus, the electrogram is the most precise way of understanding how the ICD sees the heart's rhythm. In fact, the ICD bases its therapeutic, diagnostic, and pacing decisions on the electrogram.

The electrogram looks different to a surface ECG, yet there are many points of similarity. Like an ECG, the electrogram illustrates cardiac activity in the form of a tracing, which describes electrical variations (usually in the form of curves or spikes) from a baseline. The electrogram is recorded from an electrode, which may be located in the atrium or the ventricle. Some ICDs allow a composite signal to be created from atrial and ventricular inputs. Different channels can provide different vantage points, but should not camouflage the events. Annotations on the programmer and printouts can facilitate orientation. For most clinicians, the transition from surface ECG to electrogram and vice versa is an easy leap. In fact, it's one they make every day, sometimes in the same session.

The programmer used in following an ICD will most likely offer a real-time running surface ECG parallel to the electrogram. These different annotated tracings provide a comprehensive all-round view of cardiac activity.

Electrograms are available real-time or stored. A stored electrogram has been frozen in time and stored in the memory of the device for subsequent download and analysis by the clinician. While stored electrograms are the mainstay of ICD follow-up, some introductory information is offered on the topic of real-time electrograms.

Real-time EGMs

Just like they sound, real-time EGMs provide a 'live' view of cardiac activity as seen by the electrodes of the ICD leads. Most ICD programmers allow considerable versatility in programming by offering options that let clinicians determine just what they want to see. Real-time ECGs can often be played simultaneously and parallel to real-time EGMs. For dual-chamber ICDs, clinicians can select atrial or ventricular electrograms. Some programmers will allow both to be displayed, or special EGMs, which may be a composite version of atrial and ventricular data.

Most programmers have a gain control button on the programmer, which should be left to an automatic or default setting when viewing real-time electrograms. Gain regulates how the signal data appear on the screen. The automatic or default setting is regulated so that signal data appear on the screen properly. Adjusting gain can distort the electrogram and should only be done under very careful consideration or with expert guidance. Sometimes another function called Update Auto Gains is available which automatically updates the gain on each waveform. This is a good automated feature to use to assure that the tracing can be viewed properly.

Annotations have grown so prevalent in device follow-up that most clinicians cannot really remember ECG interpretation without these markers. Annotations appear as letters, symbols or codes both to help clinicians navigate the strip and to show conclusively how the ICD categorized certain events.

Because annotations vary from company to company (and sometimes even by devices from a single company), it is recommended to check with either the physician's manual or a programmer screen to learn the code for a particular system. Nowadays, many programmers offer a screen with a Marker Legend or other information of this nature for fast, easy reference during programming sessions.

Since ICDs categorize cardiac events and intervals for diagnostic ('binning') and detection purposes, these annotations appear prominently on the electrogram on a Defibrillator Status line, typically uppermost above the electrogram. Bin categories should be listed here (for instance B for brady, S for sinus, T for Tach A, TB for Tach B, F for fib, and R for reconfirmation) along with information on arrhythmia detection. When the ICD has diagnosed an arrhythmia, a D should appear. DN means a diagnosis was made but no therapy was delivered (there are several possible explanations for this response). Depending on what supraventricular tachycardia (SVT) discrimination algorithms are activated, symbols indicating how Rate Branch evaluates the rate (< means V < A, while > means V > A) and Morphology Discrimination matches (X indicates a non-match while a check mark means match) will also appear. The Defibrillator Status line will also contain information on any therapies that are delivered; the annotation HV stands for high-voltage shock therapy delivery.

Below the Defibrillator Status line are numerical interval timing data, which may be color coded for rapid assessment. In St Jude Medical systems, blue numbers indicate atrial interval data while red data offer V–V timing interval data. Below the blue and red numbers are annotations and horizontal bars, graphically depicting the refractory periods (numerical data also appear below that in black). The horizontal bars may also be color coded; blue for atrial refractory timing cycles, red for ventricular. (See Figs 11.1 and 11.2.)

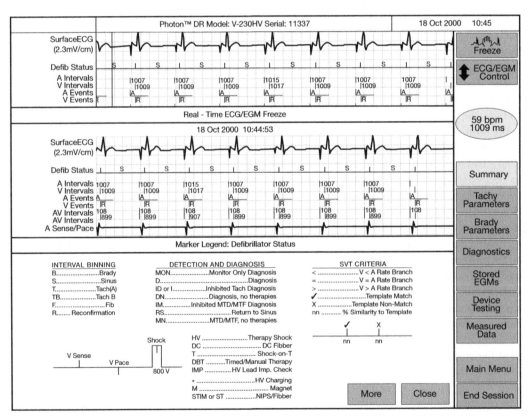

Fig. 11.1 Electrogram markers from an ICD. The surface ECG appears on the top. Below it, in parallel, is the electrogram. Annotations are listed in the legend.

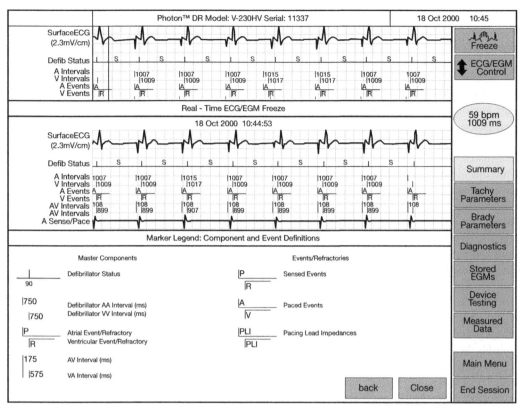

Fig. 11.2 Electrogram markers from an ICD. Some programmers provide color coding (not shown here), which allows for even more rapid visualization of what the ICD is seeing. The marker legends show event definitions.

Most programmers allow clinicians to control the markers that appear on an EGM. Other settings that can be adjusted for the electrogram include sweep speed, ECG filter, and grid. The sweep speed defines the speed of the data display and should be familiar to clinicians who work with ECGs. There may be more programmable sweep speed options for a stored electrogram than a real-time one. The default setting is 25 mm/s.

The ECG filter applies only to the surface ECG and works to help control noise that can sometimes interfere with the ECG. By turning on the ECG filter, a digital filter is activated which helps get rid of some of the stray signals and other interference ('noise') that can impair a clear ECG.

Some programmers today even allow clinicians the option of viewing the tracings against a grid or without the grid. This function is clearly a matter of clinician preference.

Real-time EGMs along with parallel real-time surface ECGs provide valuable information during most routine programming and follow-up sessions. The electrogram shows the clinician how the device is interpreting the patient's cardiac activity at that particular moment. While this is a useful feature that most ICD clinicians will use regularly, the most valuable information from an ICD generally comes from stored electrograms.

Stored electograms

The main purpose of a stored electrogram is to capture actual episode data from a patient. The stored electrogram feature allows these data to be stored in memory, so that they can be retrieved subsequently for analysis by the clinician. In order for the ICD to know what sort of episode data are desired, storage parameters for the system have to be programmed in advance. These parameters should be chosen carefully, since they determine what the ICD will record (and how it will depict it) should a tachycardia episode occur.

The size and memory constraints of the ICD impose some restrictions on just how many electrograms can be stored in memory and how much time these particular electrograms can run. Data compression techniques employed by these ICDs mean that storage times are never exact, although most manuals or specification sheets will provide good general values. ICDs can store more single-channel (atrial only or ventricular only) data than dual-channel data (atrial and ventricular data). While dual-data are generally more comprehensive and revealing, they burn up a lot of memory. For patients likely to need the benefit of more than one electrogram or longer electrograms, single-channel data may be preferable. On the other hand, for patients who do not often have episodes and for whom the clinician would like to see the most detailed data possible, dual-channel electrograms might be the better choice.

Clinicians may have the opportunity to program storage parameters for more than one electrogram. Probably the most important programming choice in setting up storage parameters is to decide the source (that is, data from which electrodes) of the electrogram. Since the ICD makes its own detection and diagnosis decisions based on information from the atrial and ventricular electrodes, the two settings A Sense/Pace (atrial electrodes) and V Sense/Pace (ventricular electrodes) are the most useful for the majority of patients. A default setting for stored electrograms is often A and V Sense/Pace.

In certain situations, it may be preferable to record electrogram data from a different source. Clinicians can program this custom EGM source using programmable options that allow them to select an anode (positive pole) and a cathode (negative pole) from a variety of choices. These choices specify the electrode (V tip and V ring, for instance, are the distal and proximal electrodes, respectively, of a bipolar lead) and even the ICD can itself (see Fig. 11.3).

While custom sources are not commonly programmed, they can provide valuable data for specific cases. By programming custom sources such as tip of the pacing or sensing lead to the distal shocking coil or ring, a near-field EGM can be created. This near-field EGM shows clinicians exactly what the device sees. This can be useful if the ICD occasionally responds in ways that the clinician could not have predicted, or if there are potential problems with sensing.

By programming far-field sources, such as setting up the electrogram to be captured from the distal shocking coil to the device can itself, a far-field EGM can be recorded which actually looks similar to a surface EGM. This provides information on possible far-field signals which sometimes can interfere with proper sensing (see Fig. 11.4).

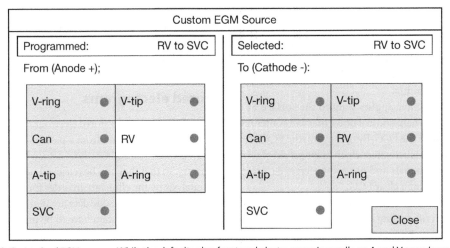

Fig. 11.3 Customized EGM sources. While the default value for stored electrograms is usually an A and V sense/pace setting, custom EGM sources can be programmed for special applications, such as recording a far-field or near-field EGM. This screen allows a variety of sources to serve as the anode (positive pole) and cathode (negative pole).

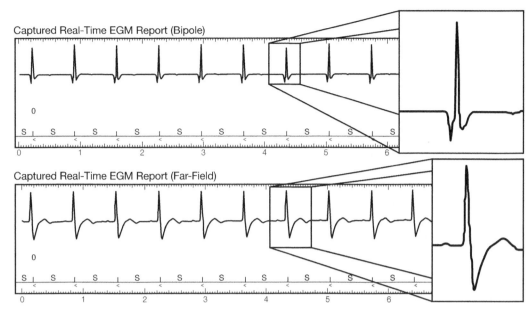

Fig. 11.4 EGMs from different sources. The sources chosen for the stored electrogram affect how the tracing will look. The top EGM is a near-field tracing, which is most similar to what the ICD 'sees.' The lower EGM is a far-field EGM, which looks more like a conventional surface ECG.

It is also possible to adjust the 'dynamic range' for stored electrogram signals. Intrinsic cardiac activity is stored in the device memory for subsequent retrieval. In order to compress and store this sort of data, it is sometimes necessary to eliminate the peaks or high points of some of the larger signals. This process of cutting signals down to size is sometimes called 'clipping.' The dynamic range determines the amplitude signal of an intrinsic P-wave or R-wave that can be stored before clipping. If you increase the dynamic range, that is, allow for larger signals before clipping occurs, the trade-off is lower resolution. On the other hand, if you want higher resolution electrograms, the trade-off is lower dynamic range. Note that the dynamic range is strictly a function of how the signals are displayed when the stored electrogram is retrieved – these changes in no way impact device sensitivity settings.

The clinician must next identify a trigger that will launch electrogram storage. The default setting is arrhythmia detection, which is defined as any time the programmed rate criteria are satisfied (for example, 12 fib intervals). As an option, the trigger can be programmed instead to diagnosis. Diagnosis is defined as a detected arrhythmia which also meets any qualifying criteria, such as Rate Branch or Mor-

phology Discrimination or other SVT discrimination algorithms. Finally, another electrogram trigger is therapy; in such cases, an electrogram is only recorded when therapy is delivered.

Although the trigger defines when the electrogram goes into action, in actual fact, the ICD is continuously monitoring cardiac activity. As a result, it is possible to program the device so that the 'pre-trigger interval' is also captured in the stored electrogram. The pre-trigger interval is defined as the time period immediately preceding the trigger, and it is programmable in seconds, usually ranging from 2 to 30 (depending on device, number of channels, and other factors). For example, if diagnosis was programmed as the trigger with a 16-second pre-trigger interval, then once the arrhythmia was diagnosed (that is, detected and meeting other criteria), the electrogram would capture the 16 seconds immediately before that diagnosis. Although there is limited electrogram storage capacity, it is generally good clinical practice to record the longest pre-trigger interval allowable. The more activity that is recorded in advance of the trigger, the greater the likelihood there is that the event that initiated the tachyarrhythmia will be recorded.

An electrogram stops storing 4 seconds after the ICD establishes sinus redetection, that is, the rate has been restored to a normal range. Many ICDs have dynamic storage capability, which means that they store electrograms of varying length and keep storing until the storage capacity is maxed out. However, sometimes rhythm disorders persist for a long time. For that reason, it is recommended that clinicians also program a maximum duration value for recording any single electrogram, usually programmable in minutes. The maximum duration simply caps the length of time that any one electrogram will be recorded. If an ICD was programmed to a 2-minute maximum duration, the electrogram would stop recording 4 seconds after sinus redetection or 2 minutes from after it started (it starts with the pre-trigger interval). Thus a 2-minute electrogram with a 16-second pre-trigger would actually store 16 seconds of pre-trigger interval followed by 104 seconds of post-trigger electrogram (16 + 104 = 120 seconds or 2 minutes).

Special events are broad terms used to refer to anything that the ICD will use as a trigger to initiate a stored electrogram (the pre-trigger interval also applies here as well). The events that can be used include typical ICD events (what the ICD defines as fib, Tach A, Tach B, tach) or when certain parameters are invoked (entry into pacemaker mode switch, PMT termination algorithm, and so on). These are individually programmable and will cause an electrogram to be stored in memory. However, because some of these events may occur frequently, the ICD will store only two such 'special event EGMs' at any given time. In addition, a special event EGM is short (16 seconds, of which 12 seconds is pre-trigger interval).

Some special EGMs are not programmable. The following special events always trigger a 16-second stored electrogram (12-second pre-trigger):

- PC shock delivery.
- Successful template verification.
- Entry into magnet reversion (this occurs when a magnet is placed over the implanted device).
- Exit from noise reversion, either atrial or ventricular channel.

Since memory is limited, most ICDs have a strategy to manage electrogram storage based on a first in/first out strategy. The idea is that the oldest electrogram chronologically is the first to be overwritten when new data comes in. Thus, clinicians reviewing stored electrograms are always examining the *latest* electrograms.

During a programming session, when an episode is being reviewed, the ICD programmer will automatically offer the opportunity to view any stored EGM related to that particular episode. Episodal diagnostics are stored and easily accessed with episode information (see Fig. 11.5).

The programmer will also offer a display button to show all stored EGMs. Scroll keys allow the material to be reviewed (see Fig. 11.6).

Stored electrograms are constantly being overwritten, so it is useful to print out any remarkable electrograms for preservation in the patient's records. When properly utilized, stored electrograms can provide valuable insight into the following (see Fig. 11.7):

- The events or mechanisms initiating tachycardic episodes.
- The patient's response to lower levels of therapy such as ATP or cardioversion.
- The adequacy of currently programmed device settings (or guidance as to how to optimize programmable parameters).
- The presence of SVTs.
- Arrhythmic episodes that resolve spontaneously.

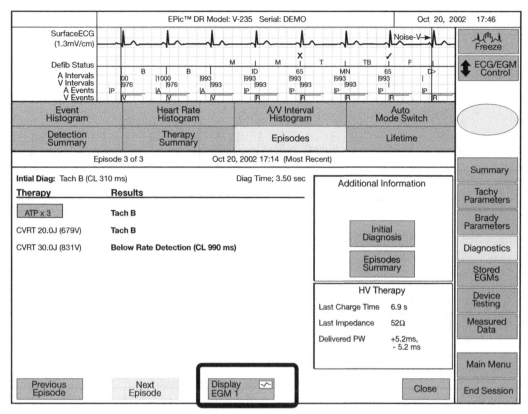

Fig. 11.5 EGM retrieval. When reviewing this particular episode on the programmer, the button at the bottom of the screen allows the clinician to go immediately to the related stored electrogram.

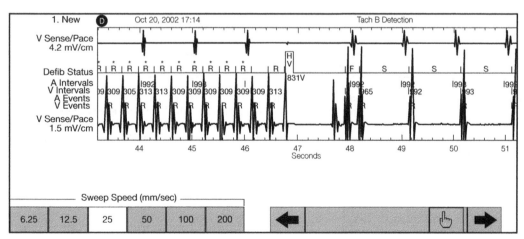

Fig. 11.6 Stored EGM. The arrows in the bottom right of the screen advance or go back to other stored electrograms in the system. Pressing the print button while the display is on screen will print out the electrogram.

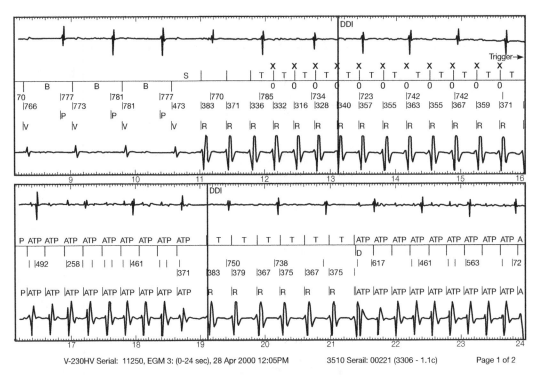

V-230HV Serial: 11250, EGM 3: (0-24 sec), 28 Apr 2000 12:05PM   3510 Serail: 00221 (3306 - 1.1c)   Page 1 of 2

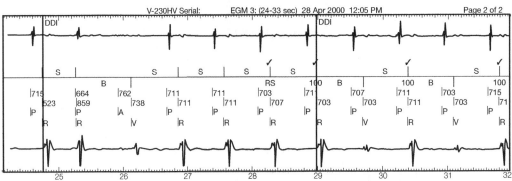

Fig. 11.7 ATP on a stored EGM. This elaborate stored EGM tells the whole story of how the ICD treated a spontaneous episode of ventricular tachycardia (VT). In the top strip, the VT was detected, which triggered the electrogram (the trigger point itself is annotated at the far right of the top strip). The ICD treated the VT with ATP (see middle strip) which slowed the VT but did not terminate it. Thus, the ICD tried ATP a second time (far right, middle strip). This converted the VT and sinus rate was restored (bottom strip).

The nuts and bolts of electrograms

- A surface ECG creates a tracing that illustrates the heart's electrical activity as it is recorded from the surface of the skin. An electrogram or EGM (sometimes called an intracardiac electrogram or IEGM) records a similar tracing but from electrodes within the heart (the ICD leads).
- An electrogram or EGM shows cardiac activity as the ICD sees it. Thus, if the ICD is behaving unexpectedly, the EGM will reveal how it records events.
- An EGM can be recorded from any of several programmable poles (anodes and cathodes) in the heart. Using the lead electrodes in the atrium and ventricle is appropriate in most cases. Far-field and near-field electrograms can be used for special diagnostic purposes.
- Near-field EGMs are closest to what the ICD 'sees,' while far-field EGMs resemble conventional surface ECGs.
- EGMs are available real-time ('live' during a programming session) or stored.
- Stored EGMs are recorded after a triggering event, typically arrhythmia detection, diagnosis or therapy. In addition, some special events may trigger a stored EGM, such as entry in mode switching or a PC shock.
- The EGM includes in its recording a certain amount of data before the trigger point. This pre-trigger interval is programmable in seconds. As a general rule, the longer the pre-trigger interval (such as 16 seconds) the more likely it is that the event which initiated the tachycardia will be recorded.
- EGMs use annotations to mark intervals, categorize events, and provide other clues to help clinicians navigate the strip. Annotations may vary by manufacturer, but there is usually a legend key or description on the programmer screen as well as in accompanying product literature.
- EGMs are stored in the memory of the ICD, which has finite capacity. Most devices have dynamic storage options, which means electrograms of varying lengths are stored until the memory is maxed out. At that point, the device starts overwriting the oldest electrograms (*first in, first out*) so that when EGMs are downloaded, only the most recent are available.
- When programming stored electrograms, clinicians often have to balance pros and cons. For instance, single-channel EGMs (ventricular or atrial only) allow for more electrograms to be stored, but dual-channel EGMs provide more comprehensive information.
- Stored EGMs can be accessed from the programmer's EGM display options or from the page where episode data are recorded.
- Stored EGMs provide a wealth of information on the mechanisms of the patient's arrhythmias, possible initiating events, response to therapy, presence of SVTs, and even how well the currently programmed parameter settings are working.

CHAPTER 12

Special features

Every new ICD on the market arrives with innovative new features and functions. While these new 'bells and whistles' are the subject of a lot of promotional activity, many clinicians only rarely use these advanced features. One reason they are not used as frequently as they ought to be involves the fact that they are new. New functions generally involve a bit of a learning curve, and most clinicians worry that they do not have time to even cover the basics, much less learn some new 'tricks' on the programmer. Another stumbling block for special features is the fact that there is no uniformity. What is available in one system may not be available in another – even from the same manufacturer. Updated features sometimes get renamed and some manufacturers offer similar functions under different names. Even an individual manufacturer may introduce a feature, rename it in a later device, or keep the name the same but re-tool how the feature works in a later product. While all of this can be frustrating to the time-crunched clinician, these features do offer real value.

Their main value resides in the fact that clinicians have very specialized tools in their toolkit for unusual or unique situations. Many special features are not designed for general all-purpose use but are simply expanded functionality and programmability for those unusual and particularly confounding cases. For that reason, it is crucial to learn in general what is available in ICDs today so that if the need arises, a clinician can put the right tools to work to help a particular patient.

For the purposes of this book, special features have been grouped into four main categories. Rather than delve into particulars on each feature (which can vary by device and manufacturer anyway), this section offers an overview. For particular special features of interest to your practice and your patients, it is recommended that you:

- Refer to the ICD manual, which generally describes all features of the device.
- Ask the manufacturer's representative for any training materials on the feature; many companies produce training manuals, booklets, pamphlets, and other materials aimed at helping busy clinicians learn product features quickly.
- Participate in seminars and other training opportunities offered by manufacturers, specialty societies, or other sources (for example, CME (continuing medical education) providers); some of these focus on particular advanced features.

Special features are available in terms of high-voltage therapy delivery, pacing, the management of atrial fibrillation, and remote patient monitoring.

High-voltage therapy delivery

There is no doubt about it: the most important thing an ICD does is deliver high-voltage defibrillation therapy to a person in danger from a potentially life-threatening ventricular arrhythmia. For patients with multiple rhythm disorders, it may be wise to program a variety of therapy options: antitachycardia pacing (ATP), as well as lower energy shocks (cardioversion) and high-energy shocks. However, one concern with this sort of programming strategy involves concern over prolonging a dangerous arrhythmia that cannot be effectively addressed with these therapeutic options. For example, what happens if a patient has a ventricular tachycardia (VT) which is first treated ineffectively with several rounds of ATP and then the device proceeds to cardioversion, which is equally ineffective. The patient could experience symptoms or worse as he or she remains in VT while the device goes through a thorough routine of trying to knock out the arrhythmia with lower energy options.

One special feature to prevent prolonged ineffective therapy is known as Maximum Time to Fib

Therapies or MTF. MTF was designed as a 'timer' that limits the amount of time the device can spend before it delivers fib therapy. In essence, MTF assures that high-energy therapy gets to the patient quickly. While MTF is designed to assure high-energy therapy, its net effect is that it allows clinicians the freedom to program ATP and cardioversion options, knowing that even if they are ineffective, the patient will still get fib therapy quickly. MTF is set nominally to 20 seconds but it can be programmed from 10 seconds to 5 minutes.

Since MTF was designed to be used in a more elaborate therapy program, it is only available when at least one SVT discriminator is used. The timer commences when the first tach interval is binned and it basically overrides continuing lower energy therapy when it times out (see Fig. 12.1).

Another concern for the clinician programming therapy is prolonged supraventricular tachycardia (SVT) activity which results in a long period of rapid ventricular response by the patient. When SVTs are detected using SVT discriminators, therapy is inhibited. But patients who experience extended spells of VT (even of supraventricular origin) may experience symptoms and require therapy. Another special feature is called Maximum Time to Diagnosis or MTD, which sets a time limit on how long the device will inhibit therapy owing to an SVT. Programmable from 20 seconds to 60 minutes, with a default setting of 30 seconds, this function allows therapy to be inhibited (because of an SVT) only until the timer expires, at which point therapy is delivered. (The feature allows the clinician to choose the first therapy delivered once the MTD expires, either tach or fib therapy, with fib therapy as the default value.)

MTD is only available in tach zones (not for fib) and at least one SVT discriminator must be turned on. The objective with MTD is to assure that patients receive the therapy they need quickly, but it also allows the clinician to program the device such that therapy can be inhibited for short runs of SVTs (see Fig. 12.2).

Pacing therapy

It is not uncommon for ICD patients to have other arrhythmias and those that do not have them when the device is implanted may develop them in the future. As such, the pacing capabilities of ICDs are growing increasingly sophisticated and many offer advanced, full-featured state-of-the-art dual-chamber pacing functionality.

Most manufacturers try to build into their top-tier ICD products the same or comparable functionality as their top pacemaker products. As such, if you are familiar with particular pacemaker device functions, you may find them transferring over to that company's ICD line.

AutoIntrinsic Conduction Search (AISC) (see Fig. 12.3) or similar features (AV Search Hysteresis) is a special function aimed at encouraging intrinsic AV conduction in a patient with a dual-chamber system by automatically and periodically extending the AV/PV delay to 'search' for native cardiac activity. The extension is programmable. The goal behind such features is to encourage intrinsic rates to prevail if at all possible. This could save on battery drain (thus possibly extending device longevity) and it definitely minimizes unnecessary right ventricular (RV) pacing.

Rate variations in pacing can occur when patients have sick sinus syndrome, brady-tachy syndrome, premature atrial or ventricular contractions, and short, self-terminating SVTs. A special feature known as Rate Smoothing is available in some devices, which helps to 'smooth out' these bumpy rates by assuring that the paced interval never varies by more than a programmed percentage of the previous R–R interval.

Atrial fibrillation

One of the most difficult clinical conditions to manage in an ICD patient (or other types of cardiac patient as well) is atrial fibrillation or AF. Since AF is the most common arrhythmia seen in clinical practice, this condition occurs frequently. Not only that, AF is a progressive disease which can occur suddenly even in patients who never had it before. As such, most ICDs need some tools for AF management.

Some ICDs offer atrial ATP options. Although atrial ATP is no sure cure of AF, it does work in some patients and should be considered. Programming atrial ATP requires some familiarity with ATP strategies and time to devote to programming the right burst stimulation patterns. Atrial ATP can be useful in the right patients.

Just as many dual-chamber pacemakers today offer mode switching, an automatic mode switch

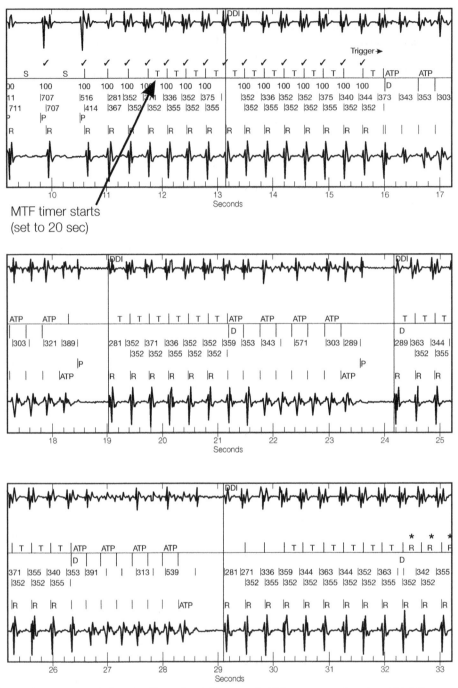

Fig. 12.1 Maximum Time to Fib Therapies. The patient is first treated with lower energy therapies which fail to convert the ventricular arrhythmia. When the MTF timer expires (in this case it is set to the default value of 20 seconds), high-energy therapy is automatically delivered, assuring that the patient does not stay too long in ventricular arrhythmia.

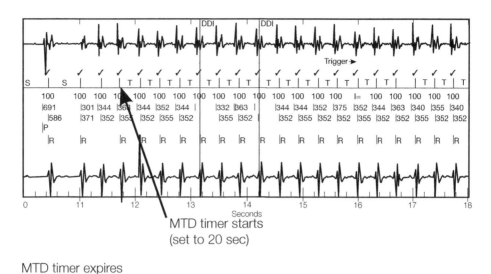

MTD timer starts
(set to 20 sec)

MTD timer expires
Tach therapy delivered

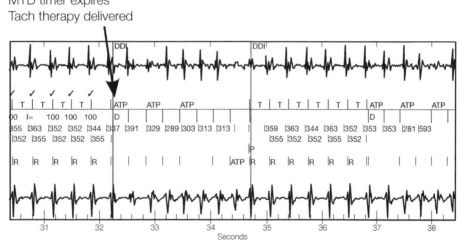

Fig. 12.2 Maximum Time to Diagnosis. The MTD timer starts when the first tach interval is binned. Here, MTD is programmed to 20 seconds. When MTD times out, diagnosis is made and therapy is delivered.

(AMS) algorithm may be available in an ICD. Essentially, AMS turns off the atrial channel in the presence of high-rate atrial activity (which is clinician-defined at the programmer) and effectively switches modes until the high-rate atrial activity is over. AMS may cause some bumps in rate, which are sometimes managed by a programmable AMS base rate, that is, a transition rate between the programmed base rate (low) and the mode switch rate (higher).

Diagnostic tools such as Cardiac Compass or AT/AF Burden Trends help report in diagnostic format how much time the patient has spent in atrial tachyarrhythmias. While these and other good diagnostic tools exist to better understand the patient's atrial rate activity over time, they can only report on *what has happened*. They cannot prevent atrial tachyarrhythmias and are best employed when some other means (pacing algorithm or drug therapy) is being used to control AF.

Pacing algorithms have long been proposed to help control AF by overdriving the atrium. It has been observed that if a pacemaker can capture and pace the atrium at a rate slightly faster than its intrinsic signal, the atrium cannot race into AF. While overdrive pacing has been around for a while (and may even be available in some ICDs), its fundamental shortcoming was that it required rapid, fixed-rate pacing of the

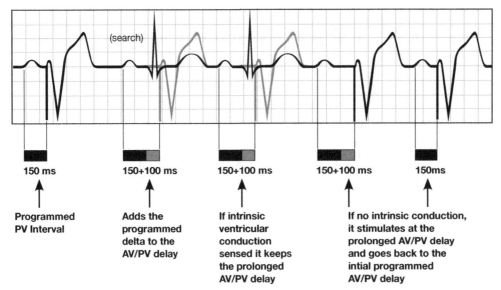

Fig. 12.3 AutoIntrinsic Conduction Search (AICS). AICS allows a programmable extension (in this case, programmed to +50 ms) to be added every 5 minutes to the AV or PV delay. This extension maximizes time for intrinsic activity to 'break through' and possibly inhibit the device. The darker lines show what would happen with a normal AV/PV delay (150 ms, in this example). The lighter lines show what happens with AICS. With AICS, there is more intrinsic (non-paced) activity.

atrium, which some patients found uncomfortable and some clinicians found nerve-wracking. The AF Suppression™ algorithm from St Jude Medical is the only clinically proven pacing algorithm designed to suppress AF by using a dynamic overdrive approach (see Fig. 12.4). The idea is that when the atrial rate started to increase, atrial pacing would overdrive the rate but only by pacing slightly faster than the patient's intrinsic rate. Sometimes this would involve rapid atrial pacing, but many times, overdrive pacing would only be modestly above the patient's own rhythm. The AF Suppression™ algorithm is automatic, requires no drugs, does not depend on patient's compliance to pharmacological regimens, and has been shown to reduce AF burden.[1] It can be programmed on and off, so it can be disabled if the patient does not need it.

Patient features

Some special features were designed for the convenience of the patient or to allow the patient greater control or awareness of the therapy.

Patient Alert is a unique feature offered by a few devices which allow the implanted device to signal the patient in the form of an audible tone in the event that something remarkable warrants medical attention. Events that might trigger a Patient Alert include out of range lead impedance values, excessively long device charge times, and sometimes low battery status. These alarms can be programmed on and off. When activating them, be sure to explain to the patient and their family what they are, since some patients may find them upsetting or may not understand what to do.

Another new twist to ICD therapy involves remote patient monitoring systems. Pacing experts have had decades of experience with transtelephonic monitoring or TTM, a type of remote monitoring system that allowed pacemaker patients to use wrist electrodes and an ordinary telephone line to report basic pacemaker function to their clinics. TTM was not very sophisticated: at most, a basic ECG and some general device parameters (usually battery status) could be downloaded. The patient just called in and performed the test over the phone. It was up to the physician's office to call the patient back if there were any unusual results.

Today, there are more elaborate systems for ICD patients. Many of them allow for considerable in-

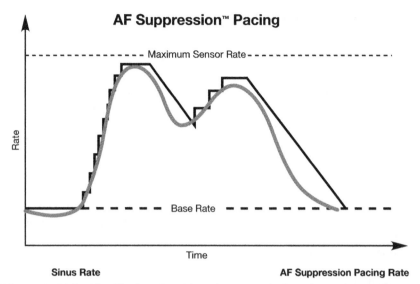

Fig. 12.4 AF Suppression™ algorithm. The dynamic atrial overdrive approach allows the overdrive pacing to occur always at a rate only slightly higher than the patient's native rate. The lighter line shows the patient's own intrinsic atrial rate while the darker line shows how the AF Suppression™ algorithm dynamically kept pace with the patient's own rate.

formation to be downloaded, including stored electrograms, diagnostic counters, and the usual parameter values. Systems may operate over the Internet or conventional phone lines. The patient may be able to talk to a real person (Housecall Plus™ remote patient monitoring system) or may respond to automated signals.

These systems work in that patients receive a transmitter, which is similar in form and function to a telephone answering machine. Patients are trained at the clinic to set up the system and transmit information, usually involving attaching wrist electrodes, making a telephone call, and then running through a simple protocol.

The utility of remote patient monitoring for ICD patients resides in its utility in treating patients immediately following therapy delivery. Many physicians encourage patients to come to the office immediately following therapy delivery. Some patients may find a shock so upsetting that they call the physician, even in the middle of the night. When an ICD patient receives a shock, everyone – the patient, the family, and the physician's office – all want to know what happened and why. A remote patient monitoring system allows a patient to send this information

to the physician before an office visit. The physician's staff (or service) may be able to interpret the results and determine that the shock was appropriate and eliminate the need and inconvenience of an office visit.

For patients who are debilitated, live far from the doctor's office, or for whom regular follow-up or post-therapy visits represent a hardship, a remote monitoring system offers the convenience of being able to get stored electrograms, diagnostic information, and other information quickly and easily. In such cases, the patient can get reassurance and medical care, even without coming into the clinic.

Most manufacturers offer or are working on remote patient monitoring systems, but at the moment, programmability via a remote system is nonexistent or drastically limited. It may be that in the future, more extensive programmability is available so that true telemedicine can be practiced for ICD follow-up.

Reference

1 Summary of Safety and Effectiveness. P8800061583 and P8300451576: St Jude Medical CRMD.

The nuts and bolts of special features

- Special features vary by manufacturer and even by device from a single manufacturer. Always check manuals and ask the device company representative for instructions.
- Most advanced features were never intended to be used for all patients. They are special tools to be used in special situations. As such, it's important to know what is available overall. You may be trying to manage a problem and have the perfect solution available in the device and not even know it.
- Some special features address therapy delivery. These manage how long the device will inhibit therapy because of an SVT (Maximum Time to Diagnosis or MTD) or how long a device will spend using less than full-energy therapies in the presence of a ventricular tachyarrhythmia (Maximum Time to Fib Therapy or MTF).
- Most ICDs offer full-featured pacemaker functionality, which can include rate response, rate smoothing, and features such as AutoIntrinsic Conduction Search (AICS) to encourage intrinsic activity and minimize the need for right ventricular (RV) pacing.
- Atrial fibrillation (AF) is the most common arrhythmia in the world and it can make ICD therapy more complicated. Many devices offer diagnostic functions to monitor AF activity, the time the patient spends in atrial tachyarrhythmias, and other counters. While diagnostic information (AT/AF Burden Trend, Cardiac Compass) is important, it only reports on the condition. The AT/AF must be managed using drug therapy or some sort of pacing algorithm.
- Many ICDs offer mode switching, which 'turns off' the atrial channel during episodes of clinician-defined high-rate atrial activity.
- The AF Suppression™ algorithm is the only clinically proven pacing algorithm shown to reduce AF burden and designed to suppress AF in device patients. It works by using a dynamic atrial overdrive pacing algorithm.
- Patient Alerts are tones or audible signals emanated by the implanted device to warn the patient about potentially dangerous conditions. If this function is available and activated, the patient requires special training so that they understand what is happening when the implanted device starts to beep!
- Remote patient monitoring systems are available for ICDs and may use conventional phone lines or the Internet. While programmability is limited (or nonexistent) patients can still send stored electrograms and diagnostic data to the clinic for analysis. This can be especially useful immediately post-therapy.
- Remote patient monitoring systems require the patient to have a transmitter and to be trained to complete the protocol using wrist electrodes and a phone line.
- Some remote patient monitoring systems offer a live person at the other end of the phone while others are more automated and direct the patient with signals.

CHAPTER 13

Diagnostics

Nowhere has the tremendous sophistication in ICD therapy been more evident than in the continuous improvement and growth of ICD diagnostics. ICDs today offer comprehensive and detailed diagnostic information, available in numeric or graphic formats, at the touch of a button. Despite the wealth of diagnostic data, many clinicians use little or none of this stored information and for understandable reasons. Extensive information can be difficult to navigate; sometimes it is difficult to know what reports to access and why. Just having a lot of information is no advantage in a clinical situation; *the right information* is needed. For that reason, clinicians can benefit enormously from spending time learning about diagnostic data options, since knowing what is available can help identify and retrieve precisely the right information when it is needed.

Diagnostic functions in a device are essentially counters, that is, they continuously monitor and record data. Some specialized diagnostic functions, like stored electrograms, have a limited storage capacity and a strategy of overwriting the oldest information (first in, first out). While it may be more difficult to max out the capacity of other, simpler diagnostic counters, it is important to erase diagnostic counters periodically so that only the latest and most relevant information is available.

Any ICD programming automatically erases the diagnostic counters (this does not apply to stored electrograms). For that reason, *when programming an ICD during a follow-up session, review and print out all diagnostic counters before you do any programming.* Once diagnostics are printed out, programming any parameter automatically resets all of the counters back to zero. Diagnostic data can also be erased by a manual programming step, but the automatic clearing with programming can be the more efficient approach. Regularly clearing out diagnostic data assures that clinicians review only device–

patient interactions since the last follow-up session.

Upon interrogation, the programmer may flag or otherwise notify the clinician that there is new or important diagnostic information in storage. This function assures that nothing is overlooked, but good clinical practice mandates that all diagnostic data be reviewed during follow-up. (See Chapter 14, *A systematic guide to ICD follow-up.*)

Just as ICDs provide both tachycardia and bradycardia therapy, they offer both tachycardia and bradycardia diagnostic functions. Diagnostic counters and functions may vary by device and manufacturer as well as by type of device (a single-chamber ICD has different bradycardia diagnostics to a dual-chamber ICD). For the most relevant details, please refer to the appropriate product manual. The following is a good general introduction.

Tachycardia diagnostics

The four broad categories of tachycardia diagnostic information captured by the ICD include detection data, therapy data, episode data, and lifetime data. Stored electrograms are also a form of tachycardia diagnostic, but were discussed in Chapter 11 and will not be addressed further here. While most clinicians find that stored electrograms along with episode data are the most useful reports for patient management, the best place to start a diagnostic data review is with detection data.

The detection summary screen shown in Fig. 13.1 provides a quick overview of what has gone on since the last time the diagnostic data were cleared (that is, the last programming session). The ICD defines an episode as any time the tachycardia detects a tachyarrhythmia. A numerical count of episodes appears on top, broken down by category (Tach A, Tach B, fib, and so on).

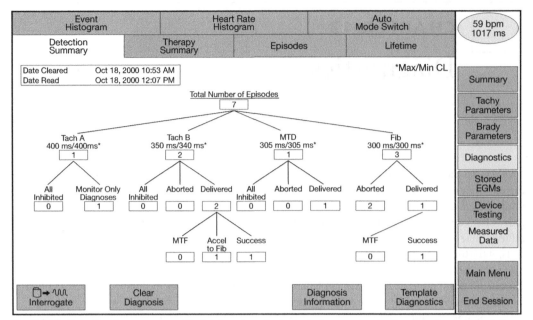

Fig. 13.1 The Detection Summary screen. The total number of episodes is shown on top, broken down in a color-coded 'tree' by category. In addition to providing the number of episodes, the maximum and minimum cycle lengths of episodes per category are stated. This example shows that the patient has had seven episodes since the last follow-up, including three episodes of VF.

In addition to revealing how many episodes occurred since the last follow-up, the breakdown of episode by category illustrates the types of arrhythmia the patient is having along with their rates. If therapy had to be delivered to address these episodes, that is stated as well. This screen also captures information on aborted therapy, inhibited therapy, and the use of certain special timing functions (see Chapter 12, Special features, for information on MTF and MTD functions).

If an episode resulted in a diagnosis of a tachyarrhythmia using the Rate Branch function (even if the diagnosis was inhibited), that information is available by drilling down one page on the programmer using Diagnosis Information. This screen contains information on any and all discriminators used in making the diagnoses (see Fig. 13.2).

The Detection Summary reports on recent modifications. If any significant changes have been made since the last time the counters were cleared (such as a Morphology Discrimination template update), that will appear in the Detection Summary. If some device-related event occurred, even if it does not require any action on the part of the clinician, it will be reported as well. An example of this might be a

report that the device detected a noise and reversion occurred.

The next destination in reviewing diagnostics is a look at the Therapy Summary, which shows information about all therapies delivered or aborted since the last time the diagnostic counters were cleared. This overview information includes shocks delivered, aborted therapies, and information on ATP (antitachycardia pacing) therapy (see Fig. 13.3).

When ATP therapy is programmed, Therapy Summary provides valuable overview data on whether ATP was actually utilized and how effective it was when deployed. Using the example in Fig. 13.3, the clinician knows that the patient has had a lot of Tach B activity (12 episodes since the last time the data were cleared) and that ATP is very often successful in terminating these events (10 out of 12 times or 83%). Furthermore, there is now documented evidence of an ATP accelerating a tachycardia, but it was a rarity (1 out of 12 events). Further, since one burst was all that was needed to successfully convert a tachycardia in 7 of the 10 successful ATP therapies, it appears that the patient responds well to ATP. Thus, a clinician can see from this screen alone that the patient has many VT episodes which

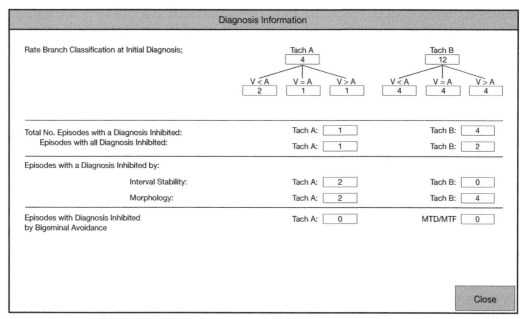

Fig. 13.2 Diagnostic information. This shows the details for all episodes that resulted in the diagnosis of a tachyarrhythmia, even if therapy was inhibited. In this example, there were four Tach A episodes and 12 Tach B episodes. However, Rate Branch excluded three Tach A episodes (V < A, V = A) and eight Tach B episodes (V < A, V = A). Interval Stability inhibited two Tach A and no Tach B therapy deliveries, while Morphology Discrimination (MD) inhibited therapy for two Tach A and four Tach B episodes.

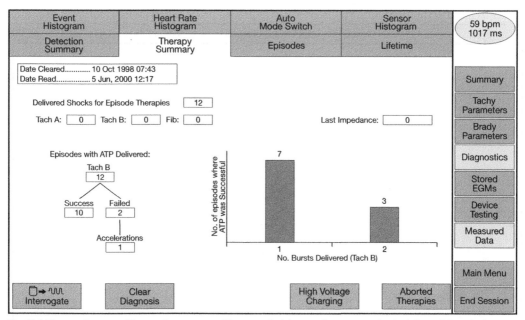

Fig. 13.3 Therapy Summary. Therapy Summary provides numerical data on the top as to shocks delivered since the last time the data were cleared. In the lower half of the screen, an ATP rate tree shows the number of times ATP was used (in this case for Tach B) with successes and failures. In this example, it shows that 1 out of the 12 ATP therapies resulted in a tachyarrhythmia acceleration. A bar chart to the right shows the number of bursts needed for successful ATP therapy; in this case, only one burst was needed to resolve tachycardia in seven instances, while in three other instances, two bursts were required. To find out more about high-voltage therapy or aborted therapies, it is necessary to press the buttons in the lower right-hand corner of the screen to go to the next pages.

can be effectively treated with ATP. While ATP does not necessarily resolve every Tach B episode, this patient has clearly been spared many shocks by having ATP activated.

While the top-level Therapy Summary screen shows how many shocks have been delivered since the last time diagnostic counters were cleared, more detailed information is available from the High Voltage Charging screen. This lists the number of shocks delivered, categorized by voltage and joule value. Manually initiated shocks, such as PC shock, shock-on-T, or DC Fibber, are also included here, but since these events are relatively rare, they will not typically be seen in the diagnostics. In the event that there have been no shocks since the last time the diagnostics were cleared, there is no screen available and the top-level screen will state that no shocks have been delivered (see Fig. 13.4).

A noncommitted ICD offers the advantage to patients that even if a diagnosis is made and the device prepares to deliver a shock, that shock can be aborted if sinus rate is confirmed. The idea behind aborted therapy is to spare patients unneeded shocks when the tachyarrhythmia resolves spontaneously. Infor-

mation on aborted therapy may also be available from the ICD. Note that a noncommitted ICD defines an aborted therapy as a situation in which charging is initiated (that is, the device prepares to shock) but the shock is not delivered. While the most common cause of aborted therapy is the detection of sinus rate, shock therapy may also be aborted if a magnet is applied over the device as it is charging or if the device goes into ventricular noise reversion mode while it is charging. Aborted therapy can be beneficial and useful to the patient, but it should always be of concern to the clinician (see Fig. 13.5).

While these broad overview diagnostics give a good idea as to how the ICD and patient have been interacting since the last follow-up session, they provide only general information: what sorts of arrhythmias were detected, what therapies were delivered, and how the patient responded. In practice, sometimes certain events require more thorough evaluation to be properly understood. For that reason, most ICDs offer episodal diagnostics. Episode diagnostics along with stored electrograms provide by far the most valuable clinical information in the follow-up setting, but it is important to start with a

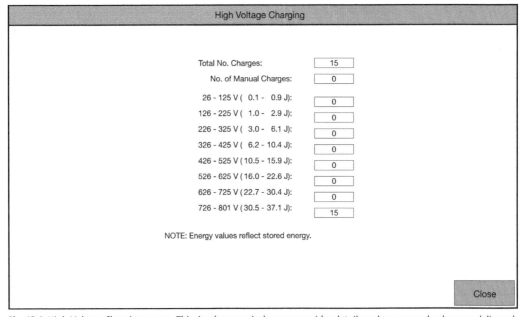

Fig. 13.4 High-Voltage Charging screen. This simple numerical screen provides details on how many shocks were delivered since the last time diagnostic data were cleared. In this case, the patient received 15 shocks, all of them initiated by the ICD (that is, 0 manually activated shocks). In this example, all of these shocks were at the highest energy level. The ICD can also be programmed to deliver 'tiered therapy,' that is, lower energy therapy for some arrhythmia categories.

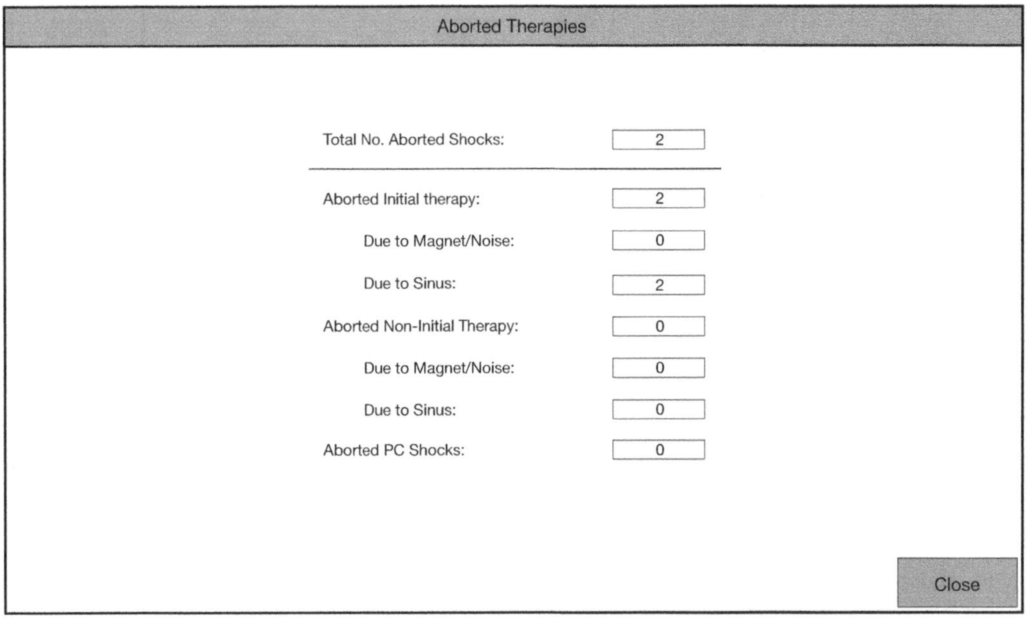

Fig. 13.5 Aborted Therapy screen. Aborted therapies are defined by the device as times when the device began charging but never delivered the shock. In a noncommitted device, therapy can be aborted when sinus rate is detected. In this example, two shocks were aborted, both for that reason. Other reasons for aborted therapy include magnet mode or noise reversion. Note that this screen subdivides aborted therapy into 'initial' and 'non-initial,' meaning the first or subsequent therapy attempts.

high-level view to know where more detailed information is needed.

Episode diagnostics store detailed records of every single episode. A limited number of episodes (for example, 60) are stored in memory and when capacity is reached, the ICD will overwrite the oldest episode with new data. (Note that programming the ICD will clear the episode diagnostics and the system starts over.) The result is that at any given time, the clinician has access to the most recent episodes in the patient's history. These episodes are identified by date and time, with the most recent episode first. But before an individual event is selected, the clinician should notice how many episodes are in memory and if there are any chronological patterns or clusters of episodes (see Fig. 13.6).

The detailed information on the episode varies by episode but includes the initial diagnosis, the type of arrhythmia, the cycle length, and what sort of therapy was used and with what results. If the episode triggered an electrogram that is still stored in memory, a button on the screen provides immediate access (see Fig. 13.7).

While most ICD diagnostics are designed to give the clinician the most recent information, one type of diagnostic is recorded and preserved over the entire service life of the device. Lifetime diagnostics capture the total number of therapy deliveries over the life of the device (grouped by energy level) as well as bradycardia information in terms of the percentage of time the device paced. Lifetime diagnostics are not only *not cleared* when the ICD is reprogrammed, they cannot be cleared, even manually. The purpose of lifetime diagnostics is to give a good overview of how much pacing the patient has received, and how many therapy deliveries have been made since the patient got the ICD. For clinicians who are seeing a new patient who has had an ICD for a while, lifetime diagnostics provides a good snapshot of how the ICD is working in the patient. Lifetime diagnostics can also give some insight into battery usage; a high percentage of pacing and multiple therapy deliveries drain the battery more than infrequent device activity (see Fig. 13.8 and Table 13.1).

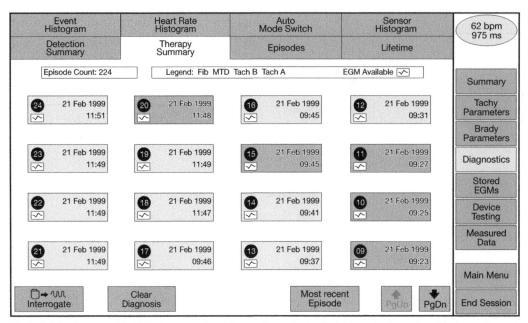

Fig. 13.6 Episodes screen. The Episodes screen shows the most recent episodes in chronological order with the most recent one first. The displays are color coded by category for easy sorting. Selecting any specific episode provides more in-depth information on that particular episode.

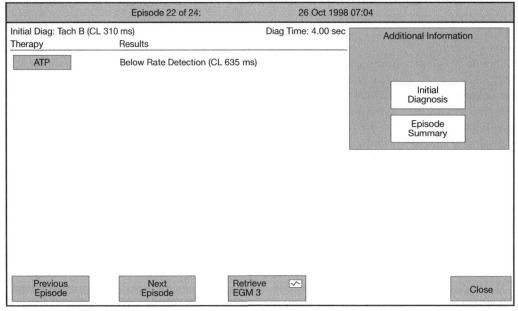

Fig. 13.7 Detailed Episode screen. The arrhythmia was diagnosed as Tach B with a cycle length of 310 ms. It took 4.00 seconds to make the diagnosis (the ICD counts this time from the first binned tachycardia interval to the point of diagnosis). This patient received ATP therapy, which extended the cycle length to 805 ms, below the rate detection level established by the device – in other words, the tachycardia was gone. The third button from the left on the bottom of the screen allows quick access to a stored electrogram of the episode.

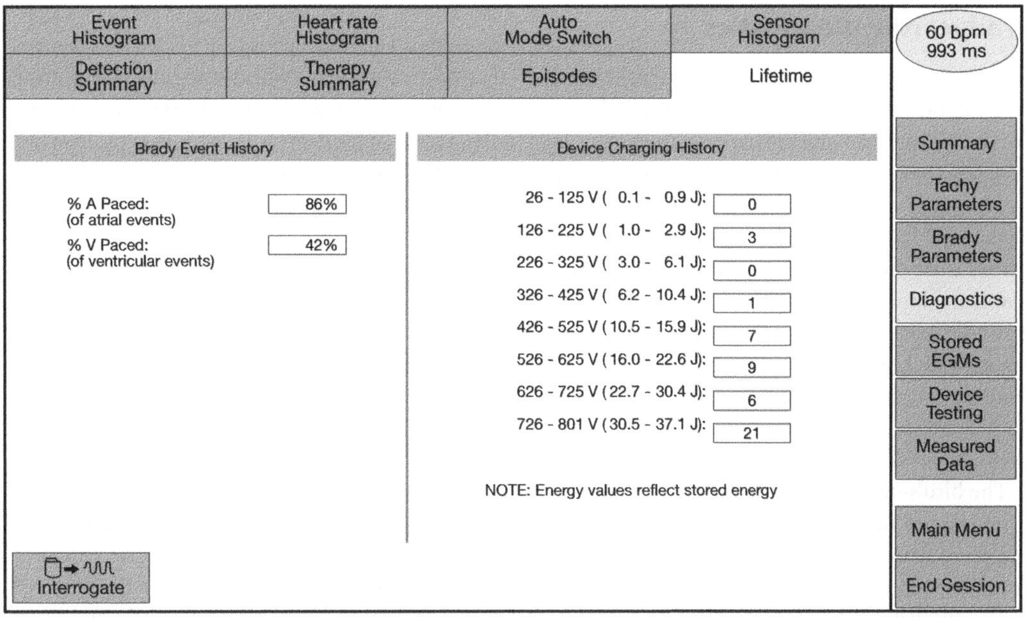

Event Histogram	Heart rate Histogram	Auto Mode Switch	Sensor Histogram	60 bpm 993 ms
Detection Summary	Therapy Summary	Episodes	Lifetime	

Brady Event History

% A Paced: `86%`
(of atrial events)

% V Paced: `42%`
(of ventricular events)

Device Charging History

26 - 125 V (0.1 - 0.9 J):	`0`
126 - 225 V (1.0 - 2.9 J):	`3`
226 - 325 V (3.0 - 6.1 J):	`0`
326 - 425 V (6.2 - 10.4 J):	`1`
426 - 525 V (10.5 - 15.9 J):	`7`
526 - 625 V (16.0 - 22.6 J):	`9`
626 - 725 V (22.7 - 30.4 J):	`6`
726 - 801 V (30.5 - 37.1 J):	`21`

NOTE: Energy values reflect stored energy

Summary

Tachy Parameters

Brady Parameters

Diagnostics

Stored EGMs

Device Testing

Measured Data

Main Menu

End Session

Interrogate

Fig. 13.8 Lifetime diagnostics. Lifetime diagnostics tells the story of the patient's interaction with the ICD over the life of the ICD. This patient has had a lot of pacing activity. He has been paced 86% of the time in the atrium, 42% in the ventricle. This indicates sick sinus syndrome and some conduction (more than half of the atrial events conducted through to the ventricle). In terms of therapy, the patient has received 21 shocks at the highest energy levels and several lower energy shocks. This appears to be a patient who needs a dual-chamber ICD! On the other hand, lifetime diagnostics do not reveal much about the patient's arrhythmias, response to therapy, or aborted therapies. For those details, other diagnostics are required.

Table 13.1 Tachycardia diagnostics

Diagnostic	What it does	When it is used	What to look for
Detection Summary	Overview of episodes by category and therapy	To get a quick snapshot of what has been going on	Has the patient had episodes? What kind? How fast were the cycle lengths? Has he or she received therapy?
Therapy Summary	Overview of ATP and shock therapy	If the patient has had therapy, this gives the details	Has the patient had ATP? Was it successful? Did it accelerate the arrhythmia?
Aborted Therapies	Overview of times when the ICD diagnosed an arrhythmia and started charging for therapy delivery but aborted the therapy	If the patient has had aborted therapies, this provides the details	Were many therapies aborted? Why were they aborted? Should the device be reprogrammed? How do aborted therapies relate to delivered therapies (were more aborted than delivered)?
Lifetime Diagnostics	Lifetime data on therapy deliveries	To check on overall device use, especially if this is a new patient or one who has had an ICD for some time	Has the patient ever received therapy? If a lot of therapy has been delivered, what is the battery status? How much pacing does the patient need? How does the history relate to what has happened since the last follow-up session?

Bradycardia diagnostics

Those who regularly work with pacemakers will find the bradycardia diagnostics on the ICD very familiar. Even those with less exposure to pacing will be able to navigate these diagnostics quickly, which are designed to show how the pacemaker function of the ICD interacted with the patient in the time period since the diagnostics were last cleared. Note that if the bradycardia pacing function in the ICD is not enabled, then no pacing diagnostics will be available. Likewise, diagnostic data will vary depending on pacing mode (single-chamber versus dual-chamber) and which features are activated (for example, mode switching).

The bird's-eye view of pacing activity in an ICD is revealed in the Event Histogram, a bar diagram of pacing activity according to type or pacing state. Pacemakers actually only do two things: they can pace (stimulate) a chamber or they can inhibit a stimulation output when they sense (detect) properly timed intrinsic activity. This means that every pacing activity is either a paced or sensed event. Using letter codes, a dual-chamber pacemaker has only four states: PR (sensed events in both chambers), PV (an intrinsic atrial beat is followed by a ventricular pacing output), AR (an atrial paced event conducts through and causes a ventricular beat) or AV (paced events in both chambers) (see Table 13.2).

The Event Histogram groups pacing activity according to these four pacing states (note that in a single-chamber ICD, only paced and sensed categories are available, since all pacing activity takes place in the ventricle only). In addition, the Event Histogram also records the number of PVEs (premature ventricular events), which are sometimes also known as PVCs (premature ventricular contractions). The ICD defines a PVE as two consecutive ventricular events without an intervening atrial event (either a sensed or a paced atrial event counts) (Fig. 13.9).

Another useful pacing diagnostic tool is the Heart Rate Histogram, a graphic and numeric display of cardiac activity grouped by rate range rather than type of activity (see Fig. 13.10). The Heart Rate Histogram gives the clinician a clear overview of where the patient's heart rate, including both paced and sensed activity. The Heart Rate Histogram captures only ventricular information (even in dual-chamber systems) so there is no confusion in the event that the patient experiences occasional episodes of atrial tachyarrhythmias. This diagnostic can help assess the chronotropic function of the heart (for example, active patients should have a suitable percentage of events at heart rates that would match their level of exertion). A large amount of high-rate activity in a sedentary patient may indicate disease progression, rapid ventricular response to an SVT, or even an arrhythmia that is sometimes called 'slow VT.' If the ICD is rate-responsive and there is a disproportionate amount of high-rate pacing, the sensor may be too aggressive and may require adjustment (this is a simple programming step).

If the dual-chamber ICD has a mode switch algorithm that is enabled, a review of the mode switch diagnostics will give an overview of how frequently this particularly algorithm was invoked. Mode switching is a special function which allows the dual-chamber pacemaker to effectively 'turn off' the atrial channel whenever it detects the presence of high-rate atrial activity. (Note that the clinician defines high-rate activity by programming the rate values; these are adjustable within broad ranges.) For example, if a

Table 13.2 Pacing states

Pacing state	Atrial activity	Ventricular activity	What it means
PR	Atrial sensed event	Ventricular sensed event	The heart is beating in the proper timing without the aid of the pacemaker
PV	Atrial sensed event	Ventricular paced event	There is intrinsic atrial activity but it is not conducting properly to the ventricles
AR	Atrial paced event	Ventricular sensed event	The atrium requires pacing (sinus node not firing properly) but the pulse conducts to the ventricle
AV	Atrial paced event	Ventricular paced event	The pacemaker is having to pace both chambers; no properly timed intrinsic activity

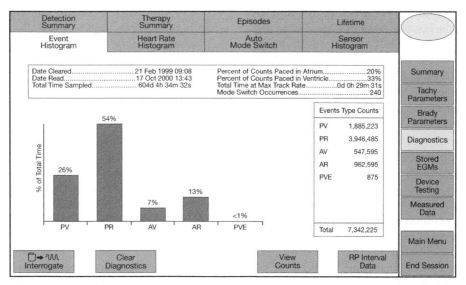

Fig. 13.9 Event Histogram. The Event Histogram captures all pacing activity since the last time the diagnostic counters were cleared in a graphic as well as numeric format. In this example, most of the activity (in fact, over a million events) was PR, that is, unpaced activity. There were also over a million PV events, in which an atrial sensed event was followed by a ventricular output pulse. In other words, an intrinsic atrial event occurred but did not conduct properly to the ventricles, so the ventricle had to be paced. This indicates that the patient relies on the pacing function of the ICD about 46% of the time (46% of the activity involved some pacing). However, the patient does have good intrinsic activity 54% of the time (PR activity) and there is intact atrial conduction (during the PR and AR events). Premature ventricular events (PVEs) are negligible at less than 1%, which is good. A large number of PVEs in a dual-chamber system would indicate the need for some troubleshooting to fine-tune device settings.

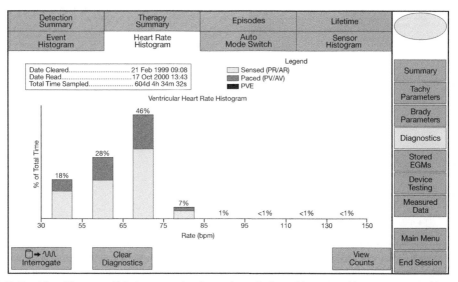

Fig. 13.10 Heart Rate Histogram. This shows paced and sensed ventricular activity grouped by rate ranges. In this example, only a small amount of activity occurred at rates between 75 and 85 beats a minute – which may be appropriate for a sedentary patient. There is certainly no alarming high-rate activity going on. Sensed activity (that is, intrinsic events) occur at varying rates, from 30 to 85 beats a minute, with most in the 65 to 75 range. Finally, there is some paced activity at the lowest range (under 55 beats a minute); the clinician should check to be sure that this is consistent with programmed settings. If not, some troubleshooting may be required.

patient experiences an atrial tachyarrhythmia, rather than let the fast atrial events possibly conduct to the ventricles and provoke a rapid ventricular response, the pacemaker simply shuts off the atrial channel temporarily, essentially changing mode (for example, an ICD that had been pacing in DDDR mode may switch to VVIR mode in the presence of high-rate atrial activity). When the atrial rate returns to normal, the mode switches back automatically to the originally programmed settings. While mode switching is an important feature, its use (particularly its frequent use) indicates that the patient is experiencing atrial tachyarrhythmias and this may require device adjustment or pharmacological therapy. At the very least, the presence of mode switch events shows that the patient is not getting the benefits of dual-chamber pacing at least some of the time. (See Fig. 13.11.)

The Mode Switch Log provides a listing of mode switch episodes with date and time of occurrence, peak rate, and duration. Stored electrograms can be set to capture entry into mode switch, so if any of these episodes has an associated stored electrogram, it can be accessed and reviewed. The stored electrogram may contain information on the event that initiated the mode switch episode and will certainly provide good insight into the nature of the high-rate atrial activity (for example, the patient may have paroxysmal AF).

If a rate-responsive ICD is programmed to sensor ON, a sensor histogram will be available to show the percentage of time that the sensor was in control of the pacing rate. Sensor-driven rates mean that the sensor (typically an accelerometer) showed the patient needed more rapid pacing support than would have been provided by the programmed base rate (for example, if the base rate was programmed to 60 ppm and the sensor controlled the rate 75% of the time, that means the accelerometer indicated that the patient needed pacing at rates of about 60 ppm three-quarters of the time). The amount of sensor-driven pacing appropriate for a particular patient depends on the patient's activity level. Very active, fit, or ath-

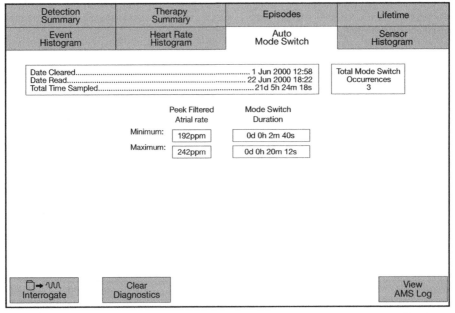

Fig. 13.11 Mode Switch screen. Mode switch diagnostics show if and how often mode switching occurred in the period since the diagnostics were last cleared. In this example, there were three mode switch occurrences. The screen also shows the minimum and maximum peak filtered atrial rate (that is, the fastest and slowest recorded events in all mode switch episodes from that period): in this case the high-rate atrial activity occurred at rates between 192 and 242 ppm (which correspond to cycle lengths ranging from 248 to 313 ms). The diagnostic also gives maximum and minimum durations of mode switch episodes. In this case, mode switching was on for 2 minutes and 40 seconds (minimum) but as long as 20 minutes 12 seconds (maximum). More detailed information can be obtained by pressing the 'View AMS Log' button at the bottom right-hand corner of the screen.

letic patients may be well served with a large amount of sensor-driven pacing, while sedentary, bed-ridden, or frail patients should have far more base rate pacing than sensor-driven pacing (see Fig. 13.12).

These pacing diagnostics will either confirm to the clinician that pacing parameter values are adequate to meet the patient's need or they may suggest that some fine-tuning is in order. They can also provide valuable information about the patient's condition and disease progression, for example, the presence of atrial fibrillation (AF) (see Table 13.3).

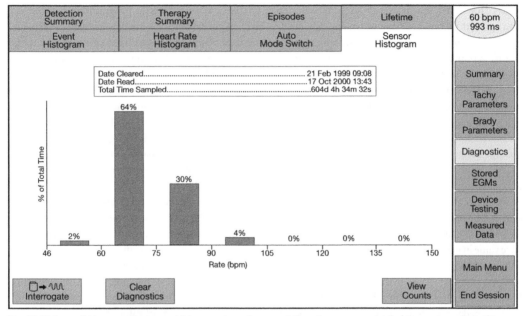

Fig. 13.12 Sensor histogram. The sensor histogram shows how much time the sensor controlled the pacing rate. In this particular example, the patient was under sensor control 64% of the time when his rate was between 60 and 75 ppm. When the patient was at rates above 75 ppm, the sensor was driving the rate up only 30% of the time. This suggests that the patient has some degree of chronotropic competence.

Table 13.3 Bradycardia diagnostics

Diagnostic	What it does	When it is used	What to look for
Event Histogram	Shows all cardiac activity by pacing state (PR, PV, AR, AV)	Used for all patients to evaluate what kind of pacing support the patient requires	Is there a lot of intrinsic activity (PR)? If there is pacing activity (any other three states), does one type predominate? Does the patient appear to have good intact conduction (PR, AR events)?
Auto Mode Switch	Shows number of mode switch occurrences and detail	For patients who have experienced mode switches, this provides detail	Are there many mode switch occurrences? What is the rate of atrial tachyarrhythmias? How long does the patient spend in mode-switched states? Does the patient have AF? (May need to see a stored 'mode switch entry' electrogram.)
Sensor Histogram	Shows amount of time the rate was driven by the sensor	For patients with rate-responsive pacing	Is the amount of sensor-driven higher-rate activity consistent with the patient's lifestyle? Does the patient appear to be chronotropically competent?

Shortcuts

Many newer models of ICDs and programmers offer some interesting programming shortcuts to help make it easier on the clinical team in charge of caring for ICD patients. Most devices today provide warning indicators when the battery voltage in the ICD drops below a certain level (typically the elective replacement indicator) or when lead impedance values (for either the pacing or the defibrillation lead) go out of range. These warnings may occur by a change in screen appearance (screen color) or involve a pop-up. Regardless of their format, these shortcut warnings offer clear explanations.

In the case of low battery voltage, it is recommended that device replacement be scheduled. Since ICD patients literally depend on these devices for matters of life and death, it is wise to arrange for prompt device replacement.

Lead impedance changes can indicate a variety of conditions. Lead impedance refers to the amount of resistance the electrical current meets within the lead. It is not a programmable value, but it is one that should be regularly monitored. While a lead impedance value in isolation may tell little about the device, any large change in impedance from one follow-up session to the next ('large' in this case is defined as 200 Ω or more) suggests that a problem is brewing. Thus, if lead impedance of the pacing lead is 300 Ω, that may fall within the normal range; but if the impedance of that same lead was 700 Ω at the previous follow-up session 6 months ago, the rapid change strongly suggests that there is some kind of lead problem.

When impedance values fall out of range or change too much from one session to the next, the best approach is to order a chest X-ray to see if there might not be some form of physical problem (insulation break, kink, tear, or lead coming loose from the generator) visible. This is covered in more detail in Chapter 15, Troubleshooting.

In addition, some programmers will immediately offer information when a device is interrogated to the effect that new stored electrograms or new tachycardia diagnostics have been recorded since the last follow-up session.

Conclusion

The world of diagnostics can be a bit overwhelming to the newcomer to ICD programming, and even very experienced ICD experts will rarely take advantage of the whole spectrum of diagnostic tools for every patient. However, a few basic points must be remembered for any effective ICD follow-up using diagnostic data:

• Always access and print out all of the diagnostic data before programming the device. Once you program anything, the diagnostic counters are cleared. (The ICD assumes you'll review diagnostics before making new programming decisions – a wise policy!)

• Always check and double-check that there are no warning messages or special information on screen. Programmers from various manufacturers are different, so you may have to 'search' a bit when working with an unfamiliar programmer.

• If there are any alerts that new stored electrograms or information is available, access and print them, if they appear to be of interest.

• Take advantage of summarized diagnostic overviews to get the big picture before drilling down into detail.

• Stored electrograms probably contain the most clinically worthwhile information, but they should be reviewed only after you've gotten the big picture to put them in proper context.

• Document everything. When in doubt, print it out!

The nuts and bolts of diagnostics

- Diagnostics provide information on how the patient and ICD have interacted over time and should be evaluated before programming the ICD in a follow-up session.
- Programming the ICD automatically erases all diagnostics, so access and print out all diagnostics of interest before programming.
- There are four main types of tachycardia diagnostics: detection data (what was detected), therapy data (what therapies were delivered or aborted), episode data (episodes by category), and lifetime data (therapy and pacing activity over the life of the device).
- The high-level overview of tachycardia performance is the detection data screen. However, clinicians often need to drill down to more detail to get the information needed to make programming or other clinical decisions.
- Therapy summary data can show if ATP options have been used and how effective they were. If a patient experiences VTs that can be successfully terminated by ATP, this can spare the patient some painful and distressing shocks.
- Lifetime diagnostics show pacing activity (in terms of percentage of time paced) and tachycardia therapy delivery over the life of the device. Unlike other diagnostic data, lifetime data cannot be erased.
- There are only four possible pacing states for a dual-chamber ICD and they are PR, PV, AR, and AV; where P is a sensed atrial event, R is a sensed ventricular event, A is a paced atrial event, and V is a paced ventricular event. The Event Histogram captures pacing activity broken down by pacing state.
- The heart rate histogram captures cardiac information grouped by rate ranges.
- The mode switch diagnostic function captures information on mode switch occurrences, duration, and the peak rate. If a stored electrogram is triggered by entry into mode switch, that data may be available as well.
- The sensor histogram shows the amount of time the paced rate was under sensor control, grouped by rate ranges.
- Modern devices and programmers sometimes offer special warning screens or pop-ups to alert the clinician to important events, such as low battery status or an out of range lead impedance value.
- Stored electrograms, covered in Chapter 11, are actually a form of diagnostic data and often provide a wealth of clinical information.
- When in doubt, print it out!

CHAPTER 14

A systematic guide to ICD follow-up

The first time an ICD is programmed usually occurs either at or immediately following implantation. After that, regular follow-up visits are recommended, usually every 1–4 months. For chronic implants in stable patients, many follow-up sessions will be mere check-ups and will not require any special reprogramming. On the other hand, problems uncovered in follow-up can be addressed and possibly even pre-empted by timely reprogramming steps.

These follow-up sessions are designed to make sure that both patient and device are doing well and interacting appropriately. While follow-up becomes a routine part of life for the ICD patient (and for the clinicians who treat them), in actuality, follow-up is a vital procedure with multiple goals and objectives, all pointing toward successful ICD therapy. The goals of ICD follow-up are:

- To assure that the patient is protected from life-threatening ventricular tachyarrhythmias.
- To verify that the ICD is functioning properly.
- To fine-tune ICD parameter values to assure optimal clinical therapy for the patient and the most efficient (not wasteful) settings for the device.
- To predict the need for possible interventions, including device replacement (battery end-of-service) or changes in patient's condition that could require device adjustment, drug therapy, other procedures, and so on.
- To minimize complications for the patient.
- To keep track of patients, answer their questions, provide reassurance and education.
- To maintain ICD system records.

The goals of ICD therapy are lofty, but actual follow-up tends to become a rote process of scheduling, tests, and documentation. For this reason, it is important for clinicians to develop a systematic approach to ICD follow-up. A system assures that no step is ever inadvertently omitted or overlooked. A system assures that all tests and procedures are properly handled and documented, even when the clinic is hectic. And a system also trains clinicians on the basic things to look for in a follow-up session.

The challenge to a systematic approach to follow-up is that ICD patients can be extremely different from one another. Some will be primary prevention patients who have never had a documented arrhythmia. Others may be bedridden with a host of other cardiac and other diseases complicating the picture. A few will be young, fit, and otherwise in generally good health, while some will be nearing death. Obviously, follow-up has to take the unique history, condition, and prognosis of each patient into account. But again, the systematic approach assures that no step is forgotten and no test is accidentally skipped.

Most modern ICDs have automated follow-up protocols that can be easily accessed by the programmer. Some programmers and devices even allow clinicians to set up custom follow-up protocols in such a way that clinicians can select the automatic protocol by pushing a button on the programmer. (These are some examples of why one might want more than one follow-up protocol: different doctors in one clinical setting may request different protocols; if the clinic is a center for a clinical trial, a trial protocol can be automated on the programmer for study subjects; and clinicians may want to set up a more abbreviated follow-up protocol for primary-prevention patients.)

Whether or not the automated follow-up is used, it is still critical to understand the sequence and elements of the follow-up procedure.

Interrogation

Interrogation begins any follow-up session and it is done when the programmer wand is placed over the implanted device and an interrogate button is pressed. The wand establishes telemetry with the device and the device begins to report basic information to the programmer.

Today's ICDs will often flag any new events during the interrogation. Such new events might be new tachycardia diagnostic information or a new stored electrogram. It is possible to shortcut from this screen directly to the new information. For a patient who presents after some sort of episode or therapy delivery, the new information may be all the clinician needs to conduct the session. But when conducting a complete follow-up, this information may be retrieved now (or later) but the clinician would then select an automated follow-up protocol (see Fig. 14.1).

If the battery is getting low or if the impedance values on the leads are out of range, a warning screen will appear during interrogation. These conditions – low battery and possible lead damage – cannot be addressed by reprogramming the device. The clinician must take steps to address these issues.

When the device indicates a low battery, an elective replacement surgery should be scheduled and the patient (if this is the first replacement) should be educated as to what to expect from this surgical revision. (Replacing the generator is a much faster, easier procedure than an initial implant and most of the time, it can be done on an outpatient basis.)

If there is a problem with the leads, the clinician must accurately determine the nature of that problem (chest X-rays are usually a good starting place) and possibly schedule surgery, either to reconnect leads that have pulled out of the generator or to replace leads which are damaged or broken. (Lead replacement is almost as involved a procedure as the initial implant, which should be made clear to the patient. Compromised leads are generally capped and abandoned rather than extracted. In fact, extraction should only be done with extreme caution and by a person experienced in the removal of chronically implanted leads. Additional risks to the patient are associated with lead removal.)

While custom protocols can be defined by the clinician, the choices for inclusion in this protocol compose the basics of any ICD follow-up session:
- Real-time measurements.
- Real-time ECG/EGM freeze.
- Stored EGM retrieval.

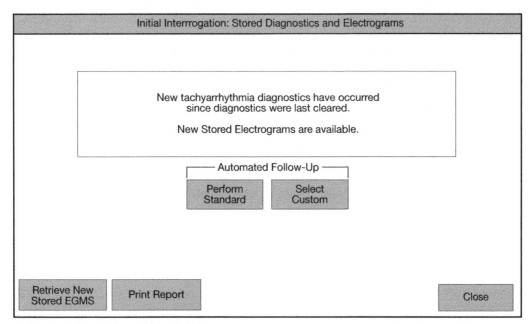

Fig. 14.1 Initial interrogation. After interrogating the ICD, the clinician learns that the device has stored some new tachyarrhythmia diagnostics and new stored electrograms since the last follow-up session. At this point, the clinician could retrieve the new electrograms and print out the diagnostics reports (buttons at the bottom left) or proceed to either a standard or custom protocol for automated follow-up.

- Capture test.
- Auto Update Morphology Template (for devices with this function).
- High-voltage lead integrity check.
- Documentation.

Real-time measurements

Real-time measurements provide some basic information on the device and patient as they are interacting at the moment the data are captured. By pressing a button, the clinician can measure the signal amplitude (height of the signal) for the patient's P-wave and R-wave, that is, for the intrinsic atrial and ventricular activity going on. The values reported here are the filtered signal amplitudes, that is, the amplitudes *the way the ICD sees them*. These values are important to compare with sensitivity settings. If the real-time filtered ventricular signal is 3.8 mV, then sensitivity has to be adjusted in such a way that a signal of this size can be 'seen' by the ICD.

If the patient is being paced most of the time, it can be difficult to measure intrinsic atrial and ventricular activity. In such cases, the clinician can take advantage of a special function called 'temporary pacing,' which allows the pacing function of the ICD to be programmed in a special way for a short duration of time. While programming the ICD clears diagnostics, temporary programming has no such effect. There are several ways to temporarily program the ICD to encourage intrinsic cardiac activity to break through (and get measured):

- The mode can be changed. If the device is pacing in DDD mode, changing the mode to VVI (no atrial pacing) will allow any intrinsic atrial activity to break through.
- The rate can be reduced. If the device is pacing at 60 ppm, lowering the rate to 40 or even 30 ppm assures that any activity faster than the temporary setting will inhibit pacing.
- Extending the AV or PV delay gives the ventricles more time to respond before a programmed output is delivered. This is useful if the patient has intact conduction but a slow ventricular response.

The pacing lead impedance values are also measured at this point (in a dual-chamber ICD, there will be an atrial and a ventricular pacing lead impedance value; in a single-chamber system, there will only be a ventricular pacing lead impedance value). Imped-ance values for a pacing lead are not adjustable, but they should be carefully monitored. The acceptable range of impedance values for a lead tends to be large, but once the impedance value is recorded (ideally, soon after implant) it should remain fairly steady. Slight fluctuations in lead impedance (say, about 5%) are normal and mean very little as regards the device–patient interaction. However, a significant change in lead impedance value (generally 200 Ω or higher) strongly suggests a lead problem, even if the new impedance value does not technically fall out of range. For example, if the pacing lead impedance value of the atrial lead was 420 Ω at the last follow-up session, but 4 months later the atrial lead impedance was measured at 742 Ω, that large change (322 Ω) indicates that something has compromised the integrity of that lead – even though 742 Ω may still technically fall within the 'normal range' of lead impedance values. Thus, while the ICD programmer will warn when impedance values go out of range (and either big increases or big drops can be warning signals), it is also important to compare the impedance values versus their previous values. For that reason, reports should be printed or impedance values noted by hand in the patient's chart.

Real-time measurements will also report actual battery voltage along with a note as to the elective replacement voltage level (typically 2.45 V).

Once the clinician has reviewed this information, pressing the Update Trends button stores this information in memory (see Fig. 14.2).

Real-time EGM

Most automated protocols allow the device to record several seconds (typically 16) of real-time electrogram before advancing to the stored EGM screen. This real-time EGM can be viewed to observe the pacing function of the ICD. The stored EGM allows the clinician to access any electrograms in memory. As a time-saving device, the stored EGM will flag any new EGMs that have been stored since the last follow-up visit. While clinicians are free to review any stored EGMs in the system, the most recently stored EGMs are generally the ones of real interest.

If no new EGM is in the system, the screen will alert the clinician that there are no new electrograms to review. For many ICD patients, it is not unusual to have no new electrograms at follow-up.

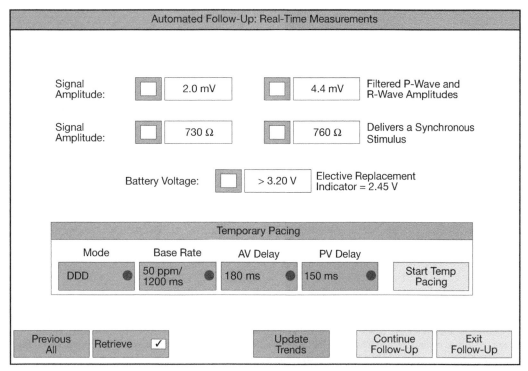

Fig. 14.2 Real-time measurements. In this example, the ICD was able to measure reasonable values for the intrinsic signal amplitudes in atrium and ventricle without requiring temporary pacing. The atrial signal was 2.0 mV and the ventricular signal was 4.4 mV. Pacing lead impedance values were 730 and 760 Ohms (Ω), which are within normal range. The ICD reports that battery voltage is greater than 3.20 V, well above the 2.45 V of elective replacement. After reviewing the information, the clinician should press Update Trends (bottom, middle) before pressing the button at the bottom right to Continue Follow-Up. Updating trends stores these real-time measurements into the device's memory.

Capture testing

The capture tests evaluate only the pacing functionality of the ICD. Since many ICD patients are pacemaker dependent or require a large degree of pacing support, the appropriate pacemaker function of the device is crucial to good therapy. Capture refers to the depolarization of the heart in response to an electrical output pulse. Without capture, the pacemaker has no effect on the heart and the patient is not getting the stimulation he or she needs. Of course, a relatively large amount of electrical energy assures that a pacing output will reliably capture the heart. The problem with this approach is that using high-output pacing pulses to providing pacing support can waste energy. Thus, clinicians need to know the capture threshold, that is, the smallest amount of energy that will reliably and consistently capture the heart. In order to accommodate possible variations in the capture threshold (capture thresholds are not stable, but vary over the course of a day, with time, disease progression, medications, and other factors), clinicians program a 'safety margin' or extra incremental amount of energy on top of the capture threshold to be sure that the capture threshold is sufficient to capture the heart over time.

Since capture thresholds can vary and since many of the causes of variations seem to describe ICD patients (disease progression, drugs), it is wise to check capture thresholds during each follow-up. There are two ways to run a capture threshold test: manually (the clinician programs the steps by hand) or semi-automatic (most of the test progresses automatically with occasional programming by hand required). The basic principle of capture testing is to decrease the pacing output in small steps till the point that capture is lost (see Fig. 14.3).

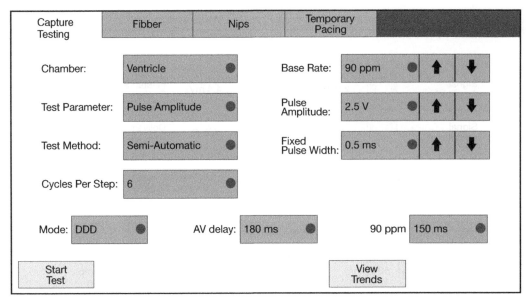

Fig. 14.3 Capture testing. Capture testing is one of the most important parts of checking out pacing function of an ICD. In this example, the clinician has programmed a ventricular capture test of the pulse amplitude using a semi-automatic test method. To test capture, the device has to be pacing. If it is not (that is, if there is a lot of intrinsic activity), pacing parameters such as mode, rate, and AV or PV delay can be adjusted on a temporary basis to assure that pacing occurs. (For example, a higher base rate or shorter AV or PV delay encourage pacing.)

When testing capture, the running real-time ECG should be used to verify pacing activity. Once pacing activity is confirmed, the parameter to be tested should be stepped down (this happens automatically in the semi-automatic test). Each time the output is reduced, the ECG should be checked to confirm that capture is still occurring. At the point that capture is lost (that is, the ICD delivers a pacing spike but there is no resulting depolarization of the heart), the test should be ended.

The programmer will capture and freeze the test electrogram. (Note that this is an electrogram, taken from within the heart by the pacing leads, rather than a surface ECG.) Using the frozen EGM and the scroll keys (arrows), the clinician can see the actual point where capture was lost. This information can be stored in the device. Knowing the capture threshold allows the clinician to program pacing output parameters appropriately. For example, if the capture threshold for the ventricle is determined to be 1 V, using the standard 2:1 safety margin for pacing, the ICD should be programmed to deliver a ventricular pacing output of 2 V. This gives the patient a safe pacing output pulse to assure consistent capture – but it is not overly wasteful of battery energy (see Fig. 14.4).

Auto Update Morphology Template

If the ICD has Morphology Discrimination, follow-up should include a step to automatically update the template. The template is a 'snapshot' of the patient's current QRS morphology at sinus rate. The update step allows the device to automatically check the currently stored template (that is, what the device 'sees' as the 'normal sinus rate' in terms of QRS shape) against the patient's current QRS morphology. If they are similar, the template is validated. If they are not sufficiently similar, the device automatically creates a new template based on the current QRS morphology.

High-voltage lead integrity check

The ICD has one lead in the ventricle through which it delivers shock therapy. This lead is known as the high-voltage lead, the defibrillation lead, or sometimes even the tachycardia lead. ICD follow-up should include a simple test to verify the proper functioning of this lead and to confirm that there is no suggestion that the lead is damaged or otherwise compromised. The device tests the defibrillation

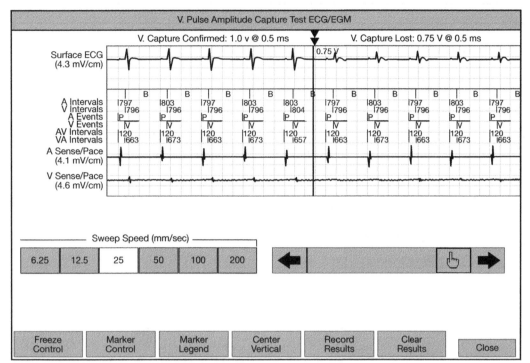

Fig. 14.4 Capture test EGM. The electrogram from a capture test has been frozen and can be scrolled (using arrow keys, bottom right) for review. The annotations show that the device captures the ventricle at 1 V but failed to capture the ventricle at 0.75 V, establishing a ventricular capture threshold of 1 V. Conventional safety margins are 2:1 or sometimes (more rarely) 3:1, which would mandate programming the ventricular pulse amplitude in this device to 2 V or possibly even 3 V.

lead by delivering a 12 V 'shock' through the shocking electrodes. While 12 V is not a large amount of energy (many pacemakers can be programmed under extreme conditions to deliver 10 V pacing outputs), most patients will be able to feel the 12 V 'shock.' Some may even find it painful and distressing. While this test is important and should be run periodically, it may not be necessary at every follow-up session.

In this test, the clinician programs the electrode configuration desired (RV to SVC/can or RV to can), initiates the test, and reviews the high-voltage lead impedance values. The patient should be properly prepared for this test and advised that he or she may feel a twitch across the chest. The lead impedance value may not match the lead impedance values reported during actual therapy deliveries; the discrepancy is due to the fact that high-voltage therapy uses a much larger amount of energy than the 12 V test output. The most important outcome of this test is whether or not the lead was able to deliver the output to the heart.

Documentation

Upon completion of the follow-up sequence, reports should be printed and put into the patient's chart. These include diagnostics, real-time measurements, capture test results, and even the parameter summary (a list of how the device is programmed). Most programmers allow clinicians to select what they want to print out and receive the copies automatically (see Fig. 14.5).

Programming

As a result of the follow-up information, it may be necessary or advantageous to adjust the parameter values of the ICD. Before this is done, it is prudent to double-check that all of the desired diagnostics have

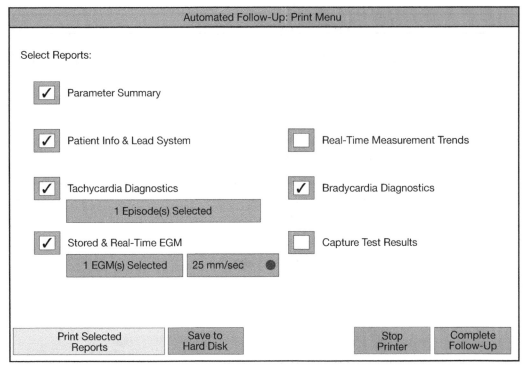

Fig. 14.5 Automated reports. After running through the automated follow-up sequence, the clinician has decided to obtain printouts of the parameter summary (how the device is programmed at the moment), patient info and lead system data, the newest tachycardia diagnostic data, the newest stored EGM, and bradycardia diagnostics. This time, the clinician has decided not to print out real-time measurements or capture test results. It is important to obtain all of this information before programming the ICD, since programming the ICD automatically clears the diagnostic counters.

been printed out, since programming automatically erases the diagnostic counters.

Programming the ICD is done using the on-screen prompts, which can also point out when programmed parameters might potentially conflict with each other. Device parameter settings are available in ranges, usually at fine incremental settings. The clinician should consult with the device manual to learn more about programmable options, default settings, and any special considerations about programming certain values. If parameter settings are changed, this should be noted in the patient's chart.

Answering the patient's questions

Part of every follow-up session should be some time set aside to address specific complaints, concerns, or questions raised by the patient. While every patient is unique and there is no way to provide blanket guidelines for all ICD patients under all circum-

stances, there are some common questions – and some good, all-purpose answers.

- *Do I have to limit my physical activities now that I have an ICD?*
  The first 2 weeks after implant, you should not raise the arm on the implant side of the body over your head. In the first 6 weeks after implant, you should avoid strenuous activity, swimming, golf, tennis, and weight lifting. After about 6 weeks, you can resume your normal activities (with physician approval).

- *Can I play all kinds of sports?*
  You should avoid contact sports (basketball or football) but not because of the exertion. Rough contact in the area of the implant could damage the device. Boxing is out, too! While doctor's orders must be taken into account, most ICD wearers can walk, jog, golf, play tennis, garden, and generally enjoy the things they used to enjoy before they got an ICD.

- *Can I go swimming?*

  While many ICD patients can and do swim, this varies by the patient. The water will not damage the ICD. You can shower, bathe, or even do water aerobics with no problem. However, patients who tend to have a lot of episodes and get shocked are urged to avoid putting themselves into situations where they might possibly have an episode in deep water – and drown.

- *What happens if I get a shock?*

  Any time you get an ICD shock, you should call your doctor. If you get two shocks in a row, that is, in a relatively short period of time, you should come into the doctor's office for a follow-up session. At the very least, the device should be interrogated and the stored EGM or diagnostics checked to see what caused the shock.

- *What if I get a whole bunch of shocks?*

  If you ever get three shocks or more in a relatively short period of time, call 911 and seek emergency help.

- *What does a shock feel like?*

  ICD patients have reported all sorts of descriptions. At one extreme are patients who receive high-voltage therapy and don't know it or aren't sure they had it. For them, shocks are very mild, maybe even unnoticeable. At the other extreme are patients who describe a high-voltage therapy delivery as like being kicked in the chest by a mule. Probably the most common response is somewhere between these two extremes. Most patients do find them painful.

- *Can I drive now that I have an ICD?*

  Do not drive a car until you have received permission from your physician. Many localities have regulations which restrict or even prohibit driving for ICD patients. The concern is that you might have an episode while behind the wheel, endangering not just your life, but the lives of your passengers and other motorists. If you have had a recent VT/VF episode, you should not drive for about 3 months. If you have frequent, recurrent episodes, you should not drive at all. This can be very inconvenient, but it is for the safety of yourself and others.

- *Can I travel?*

  If your doctor finds you fit enough, absolutely. Always carry your patient ID card and request a pat-down search at airport or security check-ins rather than walking through the metal detector. Most large airports are very familiar with dealing with pacemaker and ICD patients and will get you checked quickly and efficiently.

- *Can I use a microwave oven?*

  Yes. Most household appliances will not interfere with your ICD.

- *Should I tell my other physicians about the ICD?*

  Yes! Always tell your doctors, dentists, healthcare practitioners and others involved in your care that you have an ICD. Carry your ID card at all times. Wearing a special identifying bracelet is also highly recommended.

- *Can I still engage in sexual activity?*

  ICD patients who are healthy enough for sex can continue to have sex.

- *Do other people have these same concerns?*

  Yes. More and more Americans have ICDs and many hospitals have started support groups. These groups get together regularly to learn about their heart condition and to share their own concerns, tips, and encouragement. Many people have found ICD support groups vitally important in adjusting to ICD therapy.

Conclusion

Clinicians should approach ICD follow-up systematically to be sure that the ICD will be able to provide safe, effective therapy if and when the patient needs it. In addition, ICD follow-up can help fine-tune the device for optimal performance and be a good forum to educate the patient about ICD therapy. Today's automated follow-up protocols make follow-up quicker and easier than ever while assuring that no step is ever inadvertently overlooked. Clinicians should take advantage of follow-up sessions to be sure that the patient is adjusting well to the therapy and does not have unanswered questions.

The nuts and bolts of ICD follow-up

- ICD follow-up is intended to keep the patient safe by making sure that the device is functioning properly.
- Automated follow-up is available for newer ICDs and should be used whenever possible, because automated sequences make sure no test is ever skipped by accident.
- Follow-up can show clinicians where the device may need to be reprogrammed and alert them to possible serious conditions (lead damage, for example).
- Interrogation identifies the device and will flag the clinician about new episode data and warn them about potentially dangerous conditions (such as low battery voltage or lead impedance values that are out of range).
- Real-time measurements provide telemetered measurements of signal amplitudes, impedance values, and battery voltage.
- Pacing lead impedance values should be checked and compared at each follow-up, since a large fluctuation in values (even if those values stay within range) suggests a lead problem.
- The real-time EGM shows how the patient and device are currently interacting. Remember that the EGM shows cardiac activity exactly how the ICD 'sees' it.
- Capture testing should be performed during follow-up to be sure that the pacing outputs are adequate to consistently capture the heart.
- The high-voltage lead integrity test should be performed regularly (although perhaps not at every follow-up) to verify that the high-voltage or tachycardia lead is functioning properly.
- After follow-up, the clinician should print out reports to document the follow-up.
- No programming should occur until all diagnostics are printed out, since programming clears the diagnostic counters.
- Follow-up can be a good opportunity to educate the patient and address their questions about therapy and their 'new life' as ICD patients.

CHAPTER 15

Troubleshooting

Today's ICDs are technologically advanced, highly sophisticated, and extraordinarily reliable devices. But like any therapy, there is always the potential for problems or at least the opportunity for improvement. Problems with chronic ICD systems tend to fall into two large categories: either the device does not deliver therapy when it should have or the device delivers therapy when it is not required. Troubleshooting these problems can be approached systematically.

ICD does not deliver therapy

This is the more serious category of problems, since ICD therapy can literally be a life and death matter for patients. In the event that the patient presents in cardiac arrest or some form of cardiac distress, the first priority must be stabilizing the patient. However, if the patient presents in relatively good condition but there is evidence that the ICD has not delivered therapy when it should have, the problem needs to be determined.

Step one: Get the history of the patient and the device

Before launching any troubleshooting action, it is important to understand the patient's condition, their current drug regimens, the type and programmed settings of the device, and what the patient was doing when a 'miss' in therapy delivery occurred.

- A change in the patient's condition can mean that the previously programmed parameter settings of the device are no longer appropriate. Has the patient got worse? Have new substrates been discovered? Have new rhythm disorders (for example, atrial fibrillation) been diagnosed? In such cases, the device may have done exactly what it was programmed to do, but the patient's changed condi-

tion means that therapy was not delivered when it was needed.

- A change in pharmacological therapy can be at the root of the problem. Find out all of the medications the patient is taking, with particular emphasis on recent changes (new drugs, discontinued drugs, changes in dosage). Some anti-arrhythmic agents are known to have pro-arrhythmic qualities; taking a new anti-arrhythmic may be provoking a new arrhythmia that the ICD is not programmed to handle. Other drugs can cause elevations in DFT (defibrillation threshold), which means that even if therapy is delivered, it may not be effective.

- Verify the programmed parameters of the device and as much device history as is available. The problem may be that the device is doing exactly as it is programmed, but it is not programmed to meet the patient's need. (For example, if the device failed to deliver therapy for a ventricular tachycardia (VT) of 160 bpm that caused the patient significant symptoms but the device had a tachy rate cut-off value of 180 bpm, the device is doing exactly as it was programmed … but the programmed parameters require adjustment.) Be particularly vigilant about recent programming changes, if they are known to you.

- Find out what the patient was doing at the time. Did he or she experience any symptoms? Syncope? Was this an isolated incident or was this a recurring pattern? If they had experienced such episodes before, are they now more frequent or more severe? Find out the date and time of the event(s) for mapping the episode against device diagnostics. Since interference or magnet application can inhibit therapy, find out if the patient had been inadvertently exposed to such an environment (arc welding, high-voltage lines, industrial magnets, MRI machines, and so on). Such interference can inhibit therapy in a device that is otherwise working properly.

Step two: Get the device's side of the story

Using device diagnostics and the stored EGMs (if available), it is important to find out if the episode was captured in any way.

- Was therapy delivered during the time in question? While most patients are painfully aware of shock therapy, lower voltage therapy and antitachycardia pacing (ATP) can occur without the patient noticing anything. Just because the patient reports that no therapy was delivered does not mean it's true. If therapy was delivered, verify that therapy failed and find out what was supposed to occur. Most devices are programmed to step up therapy delivery if initial therapies fail.

- Was an arrhythmia diagnosed at the time in question? For this, the clinician needs to look at tachycardia diagnostics. Was there high-rate activity at that time? If it was captured on a stored EGM, use that to determine what arrhythmic events occurred and how the device annotated them. Was VT diagnosed? If not, why not? For example, perhaps there was high-rate activity, but it was not high enough according to the device's programmed tachycardia detection rate values. VT may have been diagnosed, but perhaps discriminators or other functions ruled that the arrhythmia was an SVT (supraventricular tachycardia) rather than a VT. If the arrhythmic event can be located and the programmed parameters were appropriate, and the ICD responded properly – it may be that the patient's episode had some other cause than something the ICD treats. For example, atrial fibrillation (AF) can produce debilitating symptoms, but it is not a rhythm disorder which the ICD treats.

- What sort of therapy is programmed? Double-check that therapy was not unintentionally disabled. (This might happen if the patient had some sort of procedure which required ICD therapy to be turned off during the operation, and it was not properly turned back on.)

- If therapy was delivered, was it adequate? For example, if the patient gets symptomatic VT that is treated by ATP (which sometimes works and

sometimes does not), it may be necessary to be sure that VT is treated more aggressively. For high-voltage therapy, find out how much energy was delivered; it may not be enough to defibrillate the heart. DFTs can change over time, even without changes in drug regimens; a 10 J shock that worked previously may no longer suffice.

- Was therapy aborted? For example, did the patient experience a nonsustained VT which produced symptoms but which resolved before therapy was to be delivered? This could be appropriate behavior on the part of the device, and something the patient might perceive as 'missed' therapy because he or she still had symptoms.

- Does the device appear to be working overall? Low battery voltage can cause the device to inhibit therapy, even if therapy is mandated.

Step three: Look for undersensing

If nothing turns up to this point, it may be that arrhythmic activity is occurring but the ICD just does not recognize it. Undersensing refers to a condition when the ICD's sensitivity setting is too high and cardiac activity passes by 'unseen.' Undersensing means that an arrhythmia will not be recognized and thus go untreated.

- Using real-time measurements, find out what the intrinsic R-wave and P-wave amplitudes are. (If the device paces constantly, use temporary pacing to lower the base rate or extend the AV or PV delay to encourage the native rate to break through.) If signals are reasonably large (1 V for atrium, 4 V for ventricle), the device should be able to sense these. If small signals are found or if stored VT/VF EGMs in memory reveal small-amplitude VT/VF episodes, it may be that during an arrhythmia, the patient's signal amplitude gets so small that the device no longer sees them.

- Verify sensing parameters. Most ICDs rely on a dynamically self-adjusting sensitivity parameter, but this can often be overridden by a manually set value. Verify that sensing is properly programmed to accommodate the patient's intrinsic signals. If sensitivity adjustments seem necessary, it is recommended to contact the technical services staff of the manufacturer or the manufacturer's representative, particularly for clinicians not very experienced in programming ICD parameter settings.

Step four: Verify ICD parameter settings

Modern ICDs are designed to offer intuitive, easy-to-navigate parameter settings, but sometimes sophisticated programming options can obscure basic therapy. Check out how the ICD is programmed.

- What is the tachycardia detection rate? Is it adequate? It may be too high for the patient's current condition, that is, the patient experiences symptoms at VT rates lower than the cut-off value.
- What sort of therapy is programmed? If ATP is programmed, how effective is ATP at breaking VT? While ATP is an important therapeutic tool in the electrical management of VT, it does not work for all patients. If lower energy shocks are programmed, how effective are they? Therapy delivery may have to be programmed to more aggressive settings.
- What sort of discriminators are in place? Was a discriminator used to inhibit therapy? If so, does the stored EGM show that this was appropriate? While SVT discrimination is an important innovation in ICD therapy, not all discriminators are appropriate for all patients. If the patient has symptomatic episodes and the device shows that discriminators inhibit therapy, those discriminators should be scrutinized and most likely turned off.

Step five: Consider the lead

The pacing and shocking electrodes of the ICD system may be at the root of a device problem.

- Check lead performance, using impedance values (real-time measurements on the programmer) and proper pacing behavior on the real-time EGM. If the device is not normally pacing, use temporary pacing to program a higher base rate or shorter AV or PV delay to encourage pacing activity. Impedance values should be in the normal range and not greatly different from their value at the last follow-up session (a great difference is commonly regarded as any change, up or down, of 200 Ω or more).
- Capture testing should be performed if there is any suspicion about pacing lead integrity. Failure to capture or great changes in capture thresholds could indicate a lead problem (or other problems, such as elevated capture thresholds).
- Perform the high-voltage lead integrity test to check that the defibrillation lead is working properly. This can be done as part of a follow-up session and does not require conscious sedation or a cath lab setting. Does the high-voltage lead seem to be working properly?
- If there are out of range impedance values, great changes in impedance values, or if the leads do not pass their appropriate tests, there may be a lead problem. The next step is to arrange a chest X-ray to ascertain if the lead is fractured, bent, broken, knicked, or otherwise compromised. (Note that not all problems will show up on an X-ray, but many will.)

Once the cause(s) of the problem is determined, the clinician should take immediate steps to correct it. These steps typically include adjusting device parameter settings, counseling the patient (for instance, to avoid high-interference environments), or replacing damaged leads.

In some cases, patients should undergo electrophysiologic (EP) testing or a procedure known as device-based testing. Device-based testing, also known as noninvasive programmed stimulation (NIPS), evaluates the patient's response to device therapy. The patient would be consciously sedated in the procedure, which often requires a short hospital stay. While this is a 'drastic' step, it can be useful if:

- There is suspicion that the nature of the patient's arrhythmic activity has changed significantly.
- The patient has not had any therapy delivery or diagnostic reports for a very long time.
- The patient complains about symptomatic episodes that the clinician cannot track down through the ICD.

During NIPS or EP testing, VF is induced in the patient and then treated with the device to verify proper response and adequate parameter settings. Because of the nature of NIPS or EP testing, it falls beyond the scope of this book. Clinicians concerned about troubleshooting a device who conclude that device-based testing is required should refer such patients to electrophysiologists or device specialists for this particular type of test.

ICD delivers inappropriate therapy

Inappropriate therapy refers to the delivery of high-voltage therapy to a patient even when the patient does not require it. While the consequences of inappropriate therapy may seem less severe than 'missing' therapy, it can still be dangerous. High-voltage therapy is distressing to the patient, and most people find shock therapy painful and upsetting. Frequent unnecessary shocks can cause tremendous psychological stress, even trauma, to the patient. Furthermore, a run of inappropriate therapy can deplete the ICD battery to the point that there is no voltage left when the patient actually requires a rescue shock. For that reason, inappropriate therapy merits the clinician's full attention.

Step one: Get the history of the patient and the device

- Why was the ICD originally prescribed? Has anything changed (new prescriptions, new conditions)? For example, has the patient recently been diagnosed with AF or some form of atrial tachyarrhythmia? Has the patient ever experienced inappropriate shocks in the past?
- Verify that the device is programmed appropriately. A very common cause of inappropriate shocks is shock therapy delivered when an SVT is detected. Are there SVT discrimination algorithms available in the device? Are they programmed or disabled? If they are programmed, are the settings appropriate?
- What is the tachy detection rate? If it is programmed too low, the device may deliver therapy when the patient is not symptomatic (for instance, the cut-off rate is programmed to 160 bpm but the patient tolerates arrhythmias up to 190 bpm).
- What was the patient doing when shocks were delivered? Were they in an environment that included potential interference (metal detectors, high-voltage areas, industrial magnets)? A high-interference environment can provoke double-counting (see Step three) and trigger inappropriate therapy delivery.
- Did the patient experience any symptoms? The absence of symptoms does not necessarily indicate the absence of a real VT.

Step two: Get the device's side of the story

In the case of inappropriate therapy, the ICD will have recorded diagnostic data and a stored EGM. These are valuable tools to access to determine what the ICD 'thought' was going on – and why it did what it did.

- Did the ICD actually deliver therapy? What was the initiating event? How did the ICD diagnose the arrhythmia? What was the actual arrhythmia?
- Did the ICD diagnose the arrhythmia correctly? If it diagnosed an SVT as a VT (which is a common cause of inappropriate shock), were discrimination algorithms programmed? The clinician should evaluate the availability of discriminators and program them carefully. Evidence from an inappropriate therapy can provide valuable insight into what type(s) of discriminators would be most useful for the patient. Not all discriminators are effective in all patients.
- What sort of therapy was delivered? If high-voltage therapy was delivered in response to a 'slow VT,' is there reason to think that the patient might not be better treated with initial ATP or lower energy shocks? What sorts of arrhythmias does the patient typically experience? If the patient has multiple types of arrhythmia, is tiered therapy programmed?
- Is the device 'seeing' an arrhythmia that isn't there?

Step three: Look for double-counting

Double-counting is a sensing problem in which the ICD mis-counts ventricular activity. One form of double-counting occurs when ventricular activity as well as T-wave repolarizations are both perceived by the ICD as intrinsic ventricular events. As a result, a natural ventricular rate of 100 bpm is counted by the device as 200 bpm … a VT, because the ICD counts the QRS complex and the resulting T-wave as separate ventricular events. Double-counting can also occur if the pacing spike is counted as an intrinsic ventricular event or when extracardiac signals (such as myopotentials or muscle noise) are counted by the ICD as ventricular events, in addition to the actual intrinsic ventricular events.

- If double-counting is occurring, there should be evidence on the annotated stored EGM for therapy delivery. What is the device counting as an R-wave? Is the device double-counting T-wave repolarizations? Has the patient changed or added any drugs which affect repolarizations (for example, anti-arrhythmics)?
- Has the patient been exposed to an environment with interference, which provoked the device into misperceiving ventricular activity?

- Is the device appropriately programmed to minimize double-counting? Sensitivity and refractory periods should be assessed.
- Is the pacemaker programmed to unipolar output? This produces a larger artifact than bipolar output. If double-counting is suspected, make sure that pacing is occurring in a bipolar configuration.

Step four: Verify ICD parameter settings

Many times, careful reprogramming of the ICD will eliminate inappropriate therapy.

- Certainly much (if not most) inappropriate therapy occurs when the device delivers therapy in response to an SVT rather than a VT. Careful programming of SVT discriminators is important. If no SVT discrimination algorithms are programmed, at least some of them should be activated.
- If the ICD has Morphology Discrimination, a template update (which can be done manually) should be performed. A change in QRS morphology can allow the device to think a sinus rhythm is actually a VT.

- If double-counting could be involved, check sensitivity settings and refractory periods.
- Check pacing parameters as well. Bipolar pacing (as opposed to unipolar pacing) can minimize double-counting.
- Confirm that the tachy detection rate is appropriate. If the cut-off rate is very low, therapy may be delivered in patients who are otherwise hemodynamically stable. (For example, if the tachy detection rate is 160 bpm but the patient does not experience symptoms unless rates are 175 bpm or higher, the cut-off rate should be adjusted to minimize inappropriate therapy.)
- Does the patient experience significant atrial tachyarrhythmias with rapid ventricular response, in particular atrial fibrillation and atrial flutter? Atrial tachyarrhythmias are often progressive in nature and can occur suddenly in patients who had not experienced them previously. Increasingly aggressive atrial rhythm disorders require more aggressive SVT discriminators.

Table 15.1 provides a troubleshooting matrix.

Table 15.1 Troubleshooting matrix

Patient complains about	Possible cause	Evidence	Remedy
Syncope with no therapy	Battery low or depleted	Use programmer to check battery status	Replace ICD
	Lead damaged or dislodged	Impedance out of range, large impedance changes, failure on high-voltage lead integrity check, X-ray shows damage	Replace lead(s)
	Device inactivated	Can be caused by inadvertent programming, magnet or backup mode, reversion; seen on programmer	Activate device
	VT occurs but is below cut-off rate	Patient has symptomatic VT at rates below tachy detection rate; may be captured on EGM or diagnostics	Lower tachy detection rate
	SVT discriminators too aggressive	Patient has symptomatic VT that meets certain SVT criteria	Make SVT discriminators less aggressive or turn them off
	Sensing problem	Device is undercounting because it does not see all the signals (many VTs have low-amplitude signals)	Adjust sensing
	Bradycardia	No evidence of VT but EGM or other evidence of bradycardia without adequate pacing support	Program more aggressive pacing parameters (e.g. higher base rate)
	Noncardiac cause	Other medical tests required	Can't be fixed by adjusting the ICD!
Shock without symptoms	Patient had VT/VF but no symptoms	EGM shows appropriate therapy response to VT/VF	Counsel patient
		EGM shows shock delivered to slow or moderate VT when perhaps ATP would have sufficed	Program ATP
	SVT is perceived as VT	EGM shows shock delivered in response to an SVT; SVT discrimination algorithms may not be programmed or programmed to very liberal values	Program SVT discrimination or make SVT discriminators more aggressive
	Double-counting	EGM shows device is counting far-field signals or T-waves as ventricular events	Increase ventricular refractory period; decrease ventricular sensing
		Pacing is unipolar	Change to bipolar pacing
		Only occurs when patient is in certain high-interference environments (device is counting noise)	Avoidance of those environments
Shock(s) but symptoms persist	Elevated DFT	Evidence of appropriate shock at value that used to defibrillate patient, but arrhythmia not broken	Increase energy output
	Shock accelerates VT	Evidence of appropriate shock that accelerates arrhythmia	Increase energy output
Multiple shocks in short period of time	Electric storm, incessant VT, ineffective previous therapies	Evidence of appropriate shocks but unbroken VT/VF	Appropriate; counsel patient
	SVTs	EGM shows therapy is being delivered to incessant SVTs	Program SVT discriminators or make them more aggressive
	Double-counting	Evidence that device is double-counting T-waves or interference	Increase ventricular refractory period; decrease ventricular sensing
	Interference	High-interference environment or special situation provoked multiple therapies	Avoidance
Never had any therapy	No VT/VF	Patient reports no symptoms, no EGM or diagnostic evidence of VT/VF	Appropriate
	Inadequate programming	Patient has symptoms, EGM or diagnostics show evidence of VT/VF, device never delivers therapy	Verify HV lead integrity, battery status, parameters; may require device-based testing
	Device not activated	Programmer shows device was inadvertently or intentionally programmed off and not reset	Program on

The nuts and bolts of ICD troubleshooting

- There are two main causes for ICD troubleshooting: either the device did not deliver therapy when it should have (causing the patient to have a symptomatic episode) or the device delivered inappropriate therapy. While patients may present with these complaints, evidence of such events may also turn up from diagnostic or stored EGMs obtained in routine follow-up.
- Of these two scenarios, therapy not delivered is by far the most serious and merits the most rigorous clinical attention.
- Patients can have syncopal spells for any number of reasons that have nothing to do with the device. This should be considered when troubleshooting the device.
- Systematic troubleshooting means getting the patient's history, checking device diagnostics, checking for sensing anomalies, verifying parameter settings, and checking for possible lead problems.
- Changes in the patient's condition and drug regimen can have ramifications for their ICD therapy. Parameter settings that worked previously may be ineffective if the patient's DFT increases or if the patient suddenly develops atrial fibrillation.
- Interference or exposure to 'noisy' environments can cause the ICD to double-count (and deliver inappropriate therapy), inhibit therapy, or even inactivate the device. It is important to understand the patient's environment when symptomatic episodes occurred.
- SVT is the most common cause of inappropriate therapy delivery and can often be effectively addressed by programming SVT discrimination algorithms.
- If therapy was delivered but not effective, the patient's DFT may have changed. DFTs are not static values, so this is not unusual. In such cases, it is useful to increase the energy output of the therapy.
- If the patient gets frequent high-energy shocks

for slow VT, ATP therapy should be considered. ATP does not work for all patients, but it has been shown to be effective in managing slow VTs in some patients. The added benefit is that it spares patients high-energy shocks and potentially saves battery energy.
- VT/VF is often characterized by low-amplitude signals. Sensitivity settings have to be sensitive enough (low enough) to detect even small-amplitude signals.
- Improper programming of the ICD can cause double-counting, such as might occur when the ICD counts both intrinsic QRS complexes and the T-wave as ventricular events; programming a longer ventricular refractory period can handle this factor.
- A common cause of withheld therapy during a VT is a tachy detection rate programmed too high.
- If the lead(s) are damaged, fractured, broken, dislodged, disconnected, or if the insulation is breached, it can show up as a variety of different problems with the ICD. Such problems include no therapy delivery, inadequate therapy delivery, and improper sensing. Lead problems usually require the implantation of a new lead; the damaged lead is usually capped and abandoned in place rather than removed. Extracting a chronic lead is a very serious procedure with a high risk of life-threatening complications and should only ever be undertaken by a specialist in such procedures.
- EP testing or device-based testing may be required to evaluate how the patient and device respond to induced VT/VF. This should only be done by an electrophysiologist.
- Some device troubleshooting is fairly basic: it is not unusual that environmental noise provoked a problem, that the device was inadvertently programmed off, or that basic parameters (SVT discriminators, tachy detection rate) were not programmed or were programmed to inappropriate settings.

Glossary

ablation A surgical process to remove tissue. An AV nodal ablation removes an area of the AV node in such a way that it interrupts a bypass tract. While ablations may sometimes be done as catheter procedures, some types of ablation (the Maze procedure, for example) require open-chest surgery.

aborted therapy The process that occurs when an ICD diagnoses an arrhythmia and begins charging to deliver therapy but something prevents the discharge of the therapeutic shock. Therapy may be aborted in a noncommitted device if sinus rate is detected after diagnosis but before therapy delivery (in other words, the patient's rate appears to have returned to normal range) or by application of a magnet over the ICD or for another reason.

absolute refractory period In pacemaker timing cycles, any time period in which the device neither sees nor counts nor responds to any activity. An absolute refractory period in a dual-chamber device may be limited to a specific channel, i.e. atrial or ventricular. See **relative refractory period**.

action potential The cycle of polarization that occurs in a cardiac cell, usually described in five phases (phase 0, 1, 2, 3, 4).

adaptive Refers to several ICD parameters which are programmed to a value that automatically adjusts or adapts to some other value. For example, burst cycle lengths in ATP can be adaptive, in which case they are programmed as percentage values of the patient's current tachycardia cycle length and automatically adjust as the patient's tachycardia cycle length changes. See **fixed**.

AF Atrial fibrillation.

anion A negatively charged particle (ion).

annotations Markers or other numerical, letter or symbolic codes placed on the electrogram to help show how the ICD counts events, refractory times, and so on. Annotations are company-specific and sometimes device-specific but are usually fairly intuitive.

antitachycardia pacing (ATP) The use of programmed low-voltage stimulation to convert a tachyarrhythmia.

arrhythmia Although the Latin meaning of this word is 'without rhythm,' it commonly refers to any type of cardiac rhythm disorder, including too-rapid and too-slow rhythms.

asynchronous Describes any output pulse (low-voltage or high-voltage) which is not timed with respect to intrinsic activity in the patient's heart. Asynchronous pacing modes such as DOO and VOO pace without sensing and may be dangerous for ICD patients.

asystole The absence of cardiac contraction, sometimes called 'flatline.'

AT Atrial tachycardia.

ATP Antitachycardia pacing.

attempt In ATP, the use of a train or programmed stimulation sequence to terminate an arrhythmia.

atrial electrogram An electrogram from the ICD's atrial channel only. This is a form of single-channel EGM.

atrial fibrillation (AF) An intra-atrial reentrant arrhythmia characterized by very rapid and apparently disorganized atrial activity which often conducts to the ventricles.

atrial flutter A form of atrial tachycardia that is rapid but very regular and characterized by a sawtooth pattern on an ECGT.

atrial tachycardia (AT) A broad term for any too-fast heart rhythms originating in the atria. See also **supraventricular tachycardia.**

automated follow-up A special programmer function in modern ICDs which allows a follow-up protocol to proceed automatically or with minimal clinician intervention. In many cases, the follow-up protocol can be customized.

automaticity   The ability of certain cells in the heart to spontaneously generate electricity. Automaticity is possessed by cells in many areas of the heart. See also **triggered automaticity**.

automatic tachycardia   A too-fast heart rhythm caused by automaticity, in this case, an abnormal acceleration of phase 4 of the action potential which causes the heart to depolarize too quickly after a repolarization. Automatic tachycardias are not caused by electrical disorders and do not respond to defibrillation. They are typically attributed to metabolic imbalances, disease, myopathy, or drug toxicity. See also **triggered automaticity**.

AV delay   The pacemaker parameter which determines how much time must elapse after an atrial output and before the next ventricular output (in the absence of intrinsic activity). See also **PV delay.**

AV nodal reentrant tachycardia   A tachycardia which originates in the AV node and is caused by a reentry mechanism. AVNRT (as it is abbreviated) is a common type of atrial tachycardia.

average interval   The value determined by the average of the current interval and the immediately preceding three intervals.

AVNRT   AV nodal reentrant tachycardia.

base rate   The programmable pacemaker parameter in an ICD which determines how fast the pacemaker function will pace the heart in the absence of sensed activity. Sometimes called **programmed rate** or **lower rate limit**.

BCL   Burst cycle length.

beats per minute (bpm)   The usual way of measuring (the natural) heart rate. See also **pulses per minute**.

bin   A rate category used for counting intervals. An example of an ICD bin is the fibrillation category. Intervals that qualify as fib are counted as such in that particular bin.

binning   The ICD's activity of constantly measuring, categorizing, and counting intervals by bins.

biphasic waveform   The morphology of a defibrillation output with a positive and negative deflection with respect to baseline. Biphasic waveforms are generally more effective at defibrillation of the heart than **monophasic waveform**.

bleeding off   The ability of a capacitor in an ICD to charge (either partially or fully) and then gradually, painlessly dissipate the charge. A noncommitted ICD may have to bleed off when a shock is aborted.

bpm   Beats per minute.

bradyarrhythmia   Any type of heart rhythm disorder in which the heart beats too slowly. **bradycardia** is a synonym.

bradycardia   Any type of heart rhythm disorder in which the heart beats too slowly. **bradyarrhythmia** is a synonym.

bradycardia diagnostics   A broad category of diagnostic data which relate to antibradycardia pacing. Examples of bradycardia diagnostics include event histograms, auto mode switch diagnostics, and sensor histograms. Some electrograms may be bradycardia diagnostics (if they relate to pacing function, for example, an electrogram triggered by entry into mode switch). See also **tachycardia diagnostics.**

Brugada syndrome   A type of triggered automatic ventricular tachycardia that appears to be hereditary and is especially prevalent in some ethnicities. A genetic mutation causes triggered automaticity. It appears that Brugada syndrome responds favorably to defibrillation.

burst   1. In ATP, a sequence of two or more precisely timed output pulses. 2. In ATP, a pattern of several bursts with or without extrastimuli. In this latter usage, burst is also known as **train.**

burst cycle length (BCL)   The programmable parameter that controls how fast the ATP output pulses are. The BCL can be fixed, that is, programmed to a millisecond value corresponding to interval length, or adaptive, programmed to a percentage of the patient's current tachycardia cycle length.

bypass tract   An abnormal conduction pathway in the heart, one that allows the electrical current to 'bypass' a straightforward conduction path. A bypass tract may be caused by any number of factors, including a myocardial infarction. A bypass tract forms a branch off the main conduction pathway but then reconnects to the main conduction pathway at a later point.

can   Slang term for the ICD generator device or the outer portion (housing) of the device.

capacitance   The capacity of a capacitor. Many factors can affect how much electrical charge a capacitor can hold and discharge successfully. Since ICDs depend on the capacitor for high-voltage therapy, the component's capacitance is important. The best strategy to maintain good capacitance is to reform the capacitors periodically (either manually or using automatic functions).

capacitor An electronic component within an ICD which stores an electrical charge until it reaches the desired proportions and then discharges it all at once. Capacitors allow ICDs with low-voltage batteries to deliver large high-voltage outputs.

capacitor maintenance The process, often automatic, which periodically reforms the capacitor of the ICD by charging it to full capacity and allowing the charge to dissipate. Capacitor maintenance prevents deformation, which can negatively impact charge times.

capture The ability of a small amount of electrical energy to cause the heart to depolarize. Pacemakers work by delivering output pulses which capture the atrium and/or ventricle.

capture test A test, often part of ICD follow-up, which establishes the patient's capture threshold. A separate capture test is needed for each chamber (atrium and ventricle).

capture threshold The smallest amount of energy required to reliably and consistently capture the heart, typically determined in a capture test.

cardiac resynchronization therapy (CRT). A device-based therapy involving low-voltage stimulation of the heart from three leads: two for the ventricles and one for the atrium. The object of CRT is to help resynchronize left ventricular dyssynchrony by helping the left ventricle contract more uniformly. CRT devices may be low-voltage (CRT-P) or high-voltage with defibrillation capability (CRT-D). CRT appears to be a promising device-based treatment option for a subset of heart failure patients.

cardiomyopathy A heart condition in which the heart muscle becomes enlarged, distended, and flabby.

cardioversion 1. The application of a relatively large amount of energy (however not as large as defibrillation) to the heart in order to convert a tachyarrhythmia. Typically, cardioversion involves energy ranging from 2 to 15 joules. 2. (for ICDs only) Any therapy delivered to respond to

an arrhythmia in a tach zone, regardless of the output.

cation A positively charged particle (ion).

Centers for Medicare and Medicaid Services (CMS) The US government offices which reach coverage decisions for Medicare and Medicaid, including what sort of devices are covered for particular indications.

cephalic cutdown A method of venous access for implanting ICD leads in which the cephalic vein is identified, lifted out, and dissected to gain venous entry. This is probably the most common method of venous access used in ICD implantation.

charge time The amount of time it takes for an ICD from diagnosis to charge to full capacity and administer life-saving therapy. Charge times can vary with device age, battery status, and the state of the capacitor.

Class I indication The condition when the evidence and/or general agreement exists among medical experts that the treatment is beneficial, useful, and effective.

Class IIa indication The condition for which there is conflicting evidence and/or a divergence of opinion about the usefulness or efficacy of a procedure or treatment, but where the weight of the evidence or opinion favors the usefulness and efficacy of the procedure or treatment.

Class IIb indication The condition for which there is conflicting evidence and/or a divergence of opinion about the usefulness or efficacy of a procedure or treatment, but where the weight of the evidence or opinion does not find the treatment useful or effective.

Class III indication The condition when the evidence and/or general agreement exists among medical experts that the treatment is not beneficial, useful, and effective.

CMS The Centers for Medicare and Medicaid Services.

coil The portion of a defibrillation lead through which a high-voltage output is delivered. An ICD lead can be single coil (one coil) or dual coil (with a proximal and distal coil).

committed The characteristic of an ICD which means that it will deliver therapy after an arrhythmia is detected. See also **noncommitted**.

competitive pacing Pacing in the presence of intrinsic activity.

connector   The clear epoxy connector block on the top of an ICD, into which one or more leads plug. See also **header.**

convert   To end one type of heart rhythm and induce another. Cardioversion is the attempt to convert atrial fibrillation to a sinus rhythm. See also **terminate.**

CRT   Cardiac resynchronization therapy.

CRT-D   The therapy provided by an implantable device that offers CRT with added defibrillation capability.

CRT-P   The therapy provided by an implantable device that offers CRT in a pacemaker (low-voltage) system (no defibrillation).

current interval   The interval (time period between two consecutive ventricular events, either paced or sensed) that is occurring at the moment. ICDs measure every interval and the current interval refers to the real-time event.

DBT   Device-based testing.

DDD   A pacemaker mode which paces in the dual chambers (atrium and ventricle), senses in dual chambers, and has a dual response to sensed events (triggered output and inhibited output).

DDDR   A pacemaker mode which paces in the dual chambers (atrium and ventricle), senses in dual chambers, and has a dual response to sensed events (triggered output and inhibited output) and has rate response, usually based on an accelerometer or activity sensor.

default value   The value of a given parameter setting in the ICD that will be used unless the clinician overrides it by programming a different value. Usually the same as the **nominal value.**

defib   An abbreviation common in ICD programming for defibrillation therapy, that is, the application of high-energy shocks.

Defib off   A type of ICD device configuration in which the ICD cannot provide high-voltage therapy. Defib off might be used temporarily for a patient undergoing a surgical procedure (where an ICD discharge might be disastrous) or for patients nearing death.

Defib only   A type of ICD device configuration in which the device categorizes all cardiac activity into only two categories: NSR or Fib.

Defib with single tach zone   A type of ICD device configuration in which the device categorizes all cardiac activity into three categories: NSR, Tach, or Fib. Different therapies may be programmed for the high-rate categories.

Defib with Tach A or Tach B   The most elaborate ICD device configuration in which the device categorizes all cardiac activity as NSR, Tach A or slow VT, Tach B or fast VT, and Fib. Different therapies may be programmed for the high-rate categories.

defibrillation   The application of a large amount of energy to the heart in order to convert a dangerous ventricular tachyarrhythmia, often ventricular fibrillation.

defibrillation lead   See high-voltage lead. Also called tachycardia lead.

defibrillation threshold (DFT)   The minimum amount of energy required to reliably defibrillate the heart. Note that DFTs are not static values and may change over time, with drugs, and with disease progression.

defibrillator status line   A row of information on an annotated EGM which contains a variety of data on how the ICD bins or categorizes various events, SVT discimrination algorithms, and other information including possibly therapy delivery.

deformation   The characteristic of a capacitor in an ICD which causes it to leak stored energy because the dielectric component within the capacitor has started to decay or become distorted. Deformation can increase charge times.

delivered energy   The amount of energy, measured in joules, that the ICD is capable of sending out to the heart. Delivered energy is different from (and less than) **stored energy**, because no capacitor can deliver 100% of its charge.

depolarization   At the cellular level, the stage in the action potential during which fast sodium channels open and allow a very rapid inflow of cations so that the cell's polarity changes quickly from negative to positive. Depolarization causes the cardiac cell to contract.

detection   The ability of an ICD to identify a potential rhythm disorder by constantly sensing and classifying intervals. Detection in an ICD is not based on clinical characteristics, but rather on rate. When specific criteria for a rhythm disorder are met through detection, the device then diagnoses an arrhythmia.

detection bin   A rate counter in the ICD for

counting intervals. The ICD uses detection bins (counters) to diagnose arrhythmias.

detection zones Categories programmed for an ICD that define sinus rhythm and rhythm disorders. Examples of zones are tach (tachycardia) and fib (fibrillation).

device configuration The manner in which an ICD is set up, that is, what sort of tachycardia or fibrillation zones are established.

detection summary A type of diagnostic data which shows the total number of episodes grouped by category (Tach A, Tach B, fib, and so on).

device-based testing (DBT) A method of implant testing using the ICD itself to help induce the patient to fibrillation in order to test the device's ability to defibrillate.

DFT Defibrillation threshold.

DFT testing The procedure during ICD implantation in which VF is induced and then the ICD is used to attempt to terminate it. DFT testing is not routinely performed today.

diagnosis In an ICD, the determination based on binning as to when an arrhythmia is present. Diagnosis is related to **detection.**

diagnosis information A form of diagnostic data which shows what criteria were used by the ICD to make a diagnosis, for example, SVT discriminators.

diagnostic data ICD reporting functions, typically in the form of counters, which provide information through the programmer on how the patient and the device have interacted over time.

diastole The period in the cardiac cycle during which one chamber of the heart relaxes. The normal heart beat has an atrial diastole followed by a ventricular diastole. See also **systole.**

diastolic function. The heart's ability to rest between beats and passively fill with blood so that it can be pumped out during systole.

double-counting Inappropriate sensing in the ICD caused by counting certain nonventricular events (such as T-wave repolarizations) as ventricular activity.

dual-chamber ICD An ICD with dual-chamber pacing capability, that is, the ability to pace DDD or DDDR mode.

dual-channel electrogram An electrogram from both the ICD's atrial and ventricular channels.

Dual-channel EGMs provide the most comprehensive information but also require the most storage space in the device's memory.

dynamic range The size of the displayed EGM signal that appears on screen before the signals are 'clipped' (that is, peaks shortened). Clipping does not change sensitivity settings.

ECG filter A digital filter in the ICD system which helps get rid of stray signals or interference (noise) that can interfere with a clear ECG.

EGM Electrogram.

elective replacement indicator The point at which it is recommended to replace an ICD because the battery energy is low. When an ICD is replaced, typically only the ICD is replaced (not the leads).

electrical heterogeneity The quality of the heart which allows different cardiac cells to be at different stages of the electrical cycle at the same time. For example, the atria can be relaxing at the same moment as the ventricles are contracting; at the cellular level, this means that cells in different areas of the heart can be depolarizing and repolarizing at the same moment.

electrogram A general term for a graphic representation of the heart's intrinsic electrical activity taken from electrodes within the heart. Abbreviated **EGM.** Sometimes called **intracardiac electrogram.**

epicardial leads The early-generation defibrillation leads which consisted of mesh patches and Dacron® rubber and were sewn onto the outside of the heart in a thoracotomy. Epicardial leads (also known as **patch leads**) are still available today but are only used in special applications.

episodal pacing Curtailed or drastically reduced pacing behavior which occurs when the ICD detects a tachycardia episode.

episode Defined by the ICD as the time period initiated by the ICD detecting a tachyarrhythmia and terminated when the arrhythmia resolves spontaneously to sinus rate or is treated.

episode diagnostics A form of diagnostic data which provides detailed information on individual episodes. There is usually a top-level screen with a listing of episodes; individual events can be accessed and information on details (time of onset, initial diagnosis, cycle length, therapy response and so on).

event histogram   A form of bradycardia diagnostic which shows all cardiac activity broken down by pacing state (PR, PV, AR, AV). An event histogram may also show the number of PVEs, as defined by the ICD.

extrastimulus   A single, precisely timed pacing output pulse used in an ATP protocol.

fib zone   A programmable rate range in the ICD that defines what rhythms the ICD will detect and diagnose as ventricular fibrillation.

fixed   Refers to several ICD parameters which are programmed to a specific, absolute value. For example, a fixed burst cycle length might be 300 ms. See **adaptive**.

fixed pulse width   An ICD configuration which keeps a constant pulse width value for output and adjusts the tilt and even energy output to accommodate that setting. See also **fixed tilt.**

fixed tilt   An ICD configuration which keeps a constant tilt value for output and adjusts pulse width to accommodate variations which might occur based on system impedance. See also **fixed pulse width.**

fluoroscopy   The use of real-time X-ray images seen on a monitor to guide ICD lead placement.

gain   A setting for electrograms which regulates how signal data appear on the screen. Most gain control should be left to an automatic regulating function, since improper gain adjustment on an electrogram may distort the way the signal appears. Gain does not affect sensitivity.

guidelines   When not specifically identified, usually refers to the ACC/AHA/NASPE 2002 Guidelines for ICD implantation [available at the website acc.org].

header   The nickname for the clear epoxy connector block on the top of an ICD, into which one or more leads plug. See also **connector.**

heart failure   A complex syndrome of conditions, usually involving but not defined by compromised left ventricular systolic dysfunction. Heart failure is typically assessed using the New York Heart Association (NYHA) classification system.

heart rate histogram   A form of bradycardia diagnostic which shows a graphic and numeric display of cardiac activity grouped by rate range.

hemodynamically stable VT   A ventricular tachyarrhythmia which does not compromise the patient's cardiac output and which will not accelerate or change into a more dangerous arrhythmia.

high DFT   In clinical practice today, a 'high' DFT is any defibrillation threshold within 10 J of the maximum output of the implantable device. For example, if an ICD can deliver 32 J of energy, then any patient with a DFT of 22 J or above would be considered to have a 'high DFT.'

high-voltage lead   The lead through which an ICD delivers shocks. Also called **defibrillation lead** or **tachycardia lead.**

housekeeping current   The amount of energy (battery drain) required by the device to maintain its status, even while the device is unused in the box. All implantable devices have some level of housekeeping current and will draw on battery energy even before they are implanted.

hysteresis   A programmable pacemaker function which sets a rate somewhat below the programmed base rate, below which the device paces. For example, if a pacemaker is programmed to a base rate of 70 ppm and a hysteresis rate of 55 bpm, the pacemaker will not pace as long as the patient's intrinsic rate is 55 bpm or higher. However, should the patient's intrinsic rate fall to 54 bpm, then the base rate takes over and, in this case, would pace at 70 ppm. Hysteresis may minimize the total time a patient is paced because it allows maximum opportunity for the patient's own native rate to prevail.

IEGM   Abbreviation for **intracardiac electrogram.**

inappropriate therapy   ICD therapy, especially high-energy therapy, delivered in response to an SVT. Although the ICD is acting appropriately (that is, doing what it was programmed to do), the therapy is not appropriate for the treatment of a rapid ventricular response to an SVT.

incidence   The number of people who can be expected to develop a condition. Usually, incidence is stated for a defined population for a specific time period (typically a year). For example, the incidence of sudden cardiac death is higher in people aged 45–75 years than in people over 75.

inter   Involving both chambers. For example, an interventricular conduction disorder is one that occurs across both ventricles.

interrogation   The initial action in any follow-up or programming session, during which the programmer wand is placed over the implanted device so that telemetry between ICD and programmer can be established.

interval   The time period in milliseconds measured between two consecutive ventricular events (either paced or sensed).

Interval Stability   An SVT discrimination algorithm available in certain ICDs which discriminates based on whether or not the R–R interval is stable. If the R–R interval is stable, the ICD diagnoses VT. If the R–R interval is unstable, the ICD diagnoses SVT.

intra   Within one chamber. For example, an intra-atrial reentry tachycardia has the reentry circuit entirely within one atrium. By the same token, an intraventricular conduction disorder occurs entirely within one ventricle (although it may affect other parts of the heart).

intracardiac electrogram (IEGM)   A graphic representation of cardiac activity, similar to an ECG, except instead of being taken from the skin's surface, it is taken from within the heart through the leads of the device.

ion   A positively charged particle. See also **anion** and **cation**.

J   Abbreviation for **joule.**

joule (J)   A unit of energy, that is, the amount of energy it takes to do the work by a force of one Newton acting through a distance of one meter. ICDs often report their output values in joules.

left ventricular ejection fraction   The amount of blood (stated as a percentage) which is ejected by the left ventricle during systole (contraction). Ejection fraction values below 40% are considered compromised.

lifetime diagnostics   A form of diagnostic data captured and preserved over the life of an ICD which records how many therapy deliveries and how much pacing the ICD has delivered. Unlike other diagnostics which can be manually erased or are automatically erased by programming, lifetime diagnostics are kept over the life of the device and cannot be erased.

lithium   One of the world's lightest metals with the highest standard potential, that is, a metal with the highest energy density. Lithium is used in implantable device battery technology as the component for the anode.

lithium-iodide cell   A battery typically used in low-voltage pulse generators and sometimes used in ICDs. Lithium acts as the anode, while iodine acts as the cathode.

lithium-vanadium cell   A battery typically used in modern ICDs in which lithium acts as the anode and vanadium (a trace element) acts as the cathode.

long QT syndrome (LQTS)   A type of triggered automatic ventricular tachycardia characterized by an abnormally long QT period on the surface ECG. Long QT syndrome can be congenital or acquired and typically occurs in children and young adults.

lower rate limit   See **base rate**.

LQTS   Long QT syndrome.

LVEF   Left ventricular ejection fraction.

macro-reentry   The mechanism for a tachycardia caused by a reentry circuit contained within a larger area of the heart. Wolff–Parkinson–White syndrome is an example of a tachycardia caused by a macro-reentry circuit.

manual   The official instructions for use of an ICD, lead, programmer, software or other product of the ICD system. All such devices must be furnished with a manual (hard copy or soft copy) which provides device specifications, instructions for use, and other pertinent details on the product.

manufacturer's representative   A person who works for and can represent the company who manufactured the ICD or any other piece of equipment used in the procedure. A manufacturer's representative may be a company official, a technical service agent, or a sales representative. Manufacturers' representatives are typically present during implantation procedures as the experts on the particular device used.

mapping   The electrophysiological process of locating bypass tracts or areas suspected of involvement in arrhythmias.

maximum duration   A programmable parameter which determines the maximum length of time an EGM will be recorded for storage in memory. An EGM may also be terminated 4 seconds after sinus redetection. In the event that sinus rate is not redetected, the maximum duration parameter sets an automatic termination point.

maximum tracking rate (MTR)   The highest rate at which the pacemaker will pace the ventricle in response to sensed, high-rate atrial activity.

membrane potential   The electrical charge inside a cardiac cell.

MI   Myocardial infarction.

micro-reentry   The mechanism for a tachycardia caused by a reentry circuit contained entirely within a very small area of the heart. AV nodal reentrant tachycardia is an example of a tachycardia caused by a micro-reentry circuit.

mode   The designation, usually stated in a three to five letter code, which determines how the pacemaker function operates (chamber-paced, chamber-sensed, response to sensed activity, rate response).

mode switch log   A form of bradycardia diagnostics which lists mode switch episodes by date and time of occurrence along with information as to peak rate and duration. If related stored electrograms are available for a particular episode, they may be accessed from this page.

monomorphic VT   A type of ventricular tachycardia which originates from one area in the ventricles. Monomorphic VT typically presents as rapid but regularly (and similarly) shaped QRS complexes. See also **polymorphic VT**.

monophasic waveform   The morphology of a defibrillation output which has only a single phase with a positive deflection with respect to baseline. See also **biphasic waveform**.

morphology   The general shape of something. Different heart rhythms present different morphologies on a surface ECG.

Morphology Discrimination   An SVT discrimination algorithm available in certain dual-chamber ICDs which discriminates on the basis of the shape of the QRS complex. The tachycardia QRS complex is compared to a sinus QRS complex stored in memory as the template. Comparisons are made on a percentage basis. If the QRS morphology matches sinus (typically a 60% match is used), the ICD diagnoses SVT. On the other hand, if the QRS morphology does not match the sinus template, then the ICD diagnoses VT.

MTR   Maximum tracking rate.

myocardial infarction (MI)   The medical term for what is commonly called a 'heart attack,' in which the coronary arteries become blocked and deprive the heart muscle (myocardium) of oxygen-rich blood, resulting in the death (necrosis) of some myocardial tissue.

myocardium   The heart muscle.

navigation   The electrophysiological process of gaining access (often by catheter) to mapped areas believed to be involved in arrhythmic activity.

nominal value   The value of a given parameter in an ICD which is deemed to be appropriate for most patients. The nominal value is usually the same as the **default value**.

noncommitted   The characteristic of an ICD which means that it will abort therapy after an arrhythmia is detected if sinus rhythm is restored before the therapy can be delivered. See also **committed**.

nonsustained   Any arrhythmia that has a duration of less than 30 seconds. See also **sustained**.

nonsustained ventricular tachycardia   A short episode of ventricular tachycardia (less than 30 seconds), sometimes even just a few beats, which spontaneously converts to normal rhythm without any intervention.

normal sinus rhythm (NSR)   For an ICD, an interval that falls within a programmable rate range associated with 'normal' cardiac activity. Thus, for an ICD, NSR is actually a rate determination. In clinical practice, normal sinus rhythm not only has to be at rates appropriate for the patient's needs, the cardiac rhythm has to originate in the SA node, conduct normally through the AV node to the ventricles, and depolarize the heart normally.

NSR   Normal sinus rhythm.

NSVT   Nonsustained ventricular tachycardia.

NYHA   New York Heart Association.

NYHA classification   The New York Heart Association system of classifying heart failure patients into one of four categories (Class I, II, III or IV) depending on their symptoms and functional capacity. This is the most common way of ranking the severity of heart failure.

pacing state   A way of classifying cardiac activity in a pacemaker patient. In dual-chamber pacing, there are only four pacing states: PR, PV, AR, and AV, where P is a sensed atrial event, A is a paced atrial event, R is a sensed ventricular event, and V is a paced ventricular event.

pacing system analyzer (PSA)   A small, hand-held device which can be used during implantation to test leads.

paroxysmal AF   A type of atrial fibrillation which

starts suddenly and self-terminates. Episodes of paroxysmal AF may be of very short duration.

patch lead See **epicardial lead.**

permanent AF A type of atrial fibrillation which is chronic and unresponsive to treatment.

persistent AF A type of atrial fibrillation which occurs for longer periods of time and requires some sort of intervention, typically medication or cardioversion, to terminate.

polymorphic VT A type of ventricular tachycardia which originates from more than one area in the ventricles. Polymorphic VT typically presents as rapid and irregularly shaped QRS complexes, because the QRS complexes have different origins. See also **monomorphic VT.**

port A cavity in the ICD connector block into which a lead plugs.

port plug A stopper, typically made of silicone rubber, which can be inserted into an unused port of an ICD at implant.

post-shock pacing (PSP) A type of pacing support provided by an ICD immediately following therapy delivery, which typically uses different pacemaker parameter values than routine pacing.

ppm Pulses per minute.

pre-trigger interval The amount of electrogram stored before the trigger point of an electrogram, usually programmable in seconds. For example if a 16-second pre-trigger interval is programmed, the ICD will store 16 seconds of activity prior to the trigger. As a general rule, the longer the pre-trigger interval, the better chance there is that the event which initiated the tachyarrhythmia will be recorded.

premature ventricular contraction (PVC) In clinical practice, an intrinsic ventricular event which occurs out of normally timed sequence, specifically too early in the sequence. PVCs can trigger reentrant tachycardias. The ICD defines a PVC as two consecutive ventricular events without an intervening atrial event. See also **premature ventricular event.**

premature ventricular event (PVE) Premature ventricular contraction. While PVC is the more common term in clinical practice, many ICDs use the term PVE. See also **premature ventricular contraction.**

prevalence The number of people in a defined population who have a specific condition.

primary prevention The strategy behind the use of ICDs in patients who have not yet had their first episode of spontaneous, sustained ventricular arrhythmia or sudden cardiac arrest. The idea is to prevent the first episode of a potentially life-threatening ventricular arrhythmia.

primary prevention trial A clinical study (often a randomized clinical trial) involving the use of ICDs in patients who have not yet had their first episode of spontaneous, sustained ventricular arrhythmias. MADIT II and SCD-HeFT are examples of primary prevention trials.

programmable polarity A parameter setting in some ICDs which allows the clinician to change the positive and negative poles of a shocking vector. For example, if the RV coil is positive and the SVC coil is negative, this could be reversed to RV coil negative and SVC coil positive. See **programmable shocking vector.**

programmable shocking vector A parameter setting in some ICDs which allows the clinician to select the electrical circuit for defibrillation energy from the choices of RV to SVC/can or RV to can. See also **programmable polarity.**

programmed rate See **base rate.**

programmer A table-top proprietary computer used to program the implanted ICD.

programming wand A telemetry head attached to the programmer by a cable and which must be placed over the implanted device to establish telemetry and do reprogramming. While most telemetry wands use a cable connection to the programmer, there are wireless wands.

PSA Pacing systems analyzer.

PSP Post-shock pacing.

pulses per minute (ppm) The usual way of measuring a paced heart rhythm. See also **beats per minute.**

PV delay The pacemaker parameter which determines how much time must elapse after a sensed atrial event and before the next ventricular output (in the absence of intrinsic activity). See also **AV delay.**

PVC Premature ventricular contraction.

PVE Premature ventricular event.

R-on-T phenomenon The response that occurs when a pacemaker delivers an output pulse during the vulnerable portion of the T-wave, inducing a ventricular tachyarrhythmia.

ramp   In ATP, the function which automatically decreases each output pulse in a specific burst by the programmed ramp step. Ramps can occur only within a burst. Also called **ramp pacing, ramping**.

ramp step   The programmable value in ATP which determines the amount that each successive output will be decreased within a burst. For instance, if a 20-ms ramp step is programmed and there are four outputs in a burst starting with an output of 320 ms, the next output will be 300 ms, followed by 280 ms and 260 ms. When that burst concludes, the next burst (should one be programmed) would start again at 320 ms and then ramp down in 20 ms steps (300 ms, 280 ms, 260 ms).

rate-responsive AV delay (RRAVD)   A programmable and automatic function in the pacemaker portion of an ICD which allows the AV or PV delay to progressively shorten as the patient's rate gets faster, mimicking the behavior of the healthy heart. Note that despite its name, rate-responsive AV delay has nothing to do with sensor-driven rate response.

rate-responsive ICD   An ICD with rate-responsive pacemaker capability, that is, the ability to pace in either VVIR (single-chamber rate-responsive ICD) or DDDR (dual-chamber rate-responsive ICD) mode.

Rate Branch   An SVT discrimination algorithm available in certain dual-chamber ICDs which discriminates based on the relationship of atrial and ventricular rates. A > V is diagnosed as SVT, A = V is diagnosed as sinus tachycardia, and A < V is diagnosed as VT. Rate Branch can be even more specific when used in combination with other algorithms.

readaptation   In ATP, the ability of a burst cycle length to change automatically (adapt) with the patient's tachycardia cycle length.

real-time EGM   An electrogram that is being displayed on the programmer as it actually happens, that is 'live.' Although ICDs offer real-time EGMs, stored EGMs have more clinical utility.

real-time measurements   In an ICD follow-up session, measurements of signal amplitudes and lead impedance values taken at the time of follow-up. Real-time measurements are often taken as the first step in follow-up.

redetection   The ability of an ICD to verify that the rhythm following a therapy delivery is either normal (sometimes called sinus redetection) or if the rhythm disorder persists (sometimes called tachycardia redetection).

refractory   A general biological term for unresponsive. Cardiac cells are refractory (cannot depolarize) during phases 1, 2, and 3 of the action potential; that is, cardiac cells cannot depolarize again until they have completely repolarized.

reentrant   The adjective which refers to rhythm disorders caused by the mechanism of reentry, for example AV nodal reentrant tachycardia.

reentry   An electrophysiologic mechanism responsible for most tachyarrhythmias, including ventricular fibrillation. During reentry, an electrical impulse from the heart enters a circular substrate in such a way that the impulse travels round and round, gaining speed, and provoking a dangerous and disordered heart rhythm.

reformation   The process of improving capacitor performance by charging the capacitor completely and allowing the charge to painlessly dissipate. Reforming the capacitor improves the state of the dielectric component within the capacitor. Capacitors can be reformed automatically or manually.

relative refractory period   In pacemaker timing cycles, any time period in which the device does not respond to activity, but sees it and counts it in the diagnostic counters. See **absolute refractory period**.

repolarization   At the cellular level, the stage in the action potential following contraction of the cell during which sodium cations leave the interior of the cell and the cell gets back to resting membrane potential or its relaxed, resting state.

rescue   A therapeutic approach or strategy which saves a patient from a potentially life-threatening condition but which does not attempt to suppress that condition, alleviate symptoms, or cure the condition. Defibrillation rescues patients; it does not cure ventricular fibrillation.

rest rate   A pacemaker function which allows the pacemaker to pace at slower-than-base-rate values when the patient is asleep or resting. Some devices set rest rate based on clock time, but others use auto rest rate, based on sensor input.

risk factors   Known attributes, behaviors or other

conditions that have been associated with an increased likelihood of developing a certain condition. For example, smoking and family history of heart disease are risk factors for coronary artery disease.

RRAVD   Rate-responsive AV delay.

safety margin   The 'margin for error' when programming pacemaker outputs to assure that the device captures the heart. When programming pulse amplitude settings, the conventional safety margin is 2:1; where 1 is the capture threshold and 2 is the pulse amplitude setting of the device. Sometimes larger safety margins are recommended.

SCA   Sudden cardiac arrest.

scanning   In ATP, the function which allows the cycle length to be changed from one burst to the next. Scanning affects cycle length from burst to burst, while ramping decreases outputs within a burst.

SCD   Sudden cardiac death.

self-terminate   The ability of an arrhythmia to stop spontaneously with no outside intervention.

sensing   The ability of an ICD to detect ('sense') intrinsic cardiac activity by picking up electrical signals from the heart through the leads. The device's ability to sense is governed by the sensitivity parameters. Sensing is related to detection but detection refers to the ability not just to sense signals but to classify and count them.

sensitivity   For an ICD, the ability to recognize and respond to ventricular tachyarrhythmias. Many ICDs have 100% sensitivity, which means they do not fail to recognize and treat these life-threatening arrhythmias. See also **specificity**.

sensor   In a rate-responsive ICD, the accelerometer or other type of component which determines if the patient requires a faster paced rate. Most rate-responsive ICDs use activity sensors (accelerometers or piezoelectric crystals).

sensor histogram   A type of bradycardia diagnostic which shows how much time and at what rate ranges the sensor of a rate-responsive device was in control of the pacing rate.

shock   The nickname for high-energy therapy delivery from an ICD.

shocking vector   The path that defibrillating energy takes through the heart. For ICD patients,
the shocking vector may form a current pathway from the two coils of the defibrillating lead or from one coil of the lead and the ICD can itself.

single-chamber ICD   An ICD with single-chamber ventricular pacing capability (VVI or VVIR).

sinus redetection   The ability of the ICD to confirm that sinus activity is present in the intervals immediately following therapy delivery. When sinus rhythm is redetected, the device 'concludes' that the therapy was effective and does not continue with therapeutic interventions.

sinus rhythm   1. The rhythm of the healthy heart, driven by electrical outputs from the heart's natural pacemaker, the SA node, and properly conducted throughout the heart. 2. For ICD therapy, sinus rhythm refers to a programmable rate range that the device recognizes as sinus rhythm. What the ICD defines as sinus rhythm may not be the same as clinical sinus rhythm.

special events   Events that will trigger a stored electrogram. These are sometimes programmable (for example, entry in mode switch) or sometimes fixed (for example, entry into magnet reversion).

specificity   The ability of an ICD to distinguish between arrhythmias it ought to treat (VT/VF) and SVTs. While most ICDs with SVT discrimination offer high specificity values, 100% specificity has not yet been achieved.

stored electrogram   An electrogram which is placed in the memory of the implanted device and which can be retrieved using the programmer for subsequent analysis. Stored electrograms are a form of **diagnostic data**. Note that older ICDs may not have stored electrogram capability or may have very limited memory capacity.

stored energy   The amount of energy, measured in joules, which the ICD is capable of holding in its capacitors. Stored energy is different from (and greater than) **delivered energy**.

subclavian stick   A venous approach using a modified Seldinger technique in which the subclavian vein is punctured. This is a common method of gaining venous access for ICD leads.

substrate   An area on the heart muscle (myocardium) which becomes a viable alternate electrical pathway for the heart.

sudden cardiac arrest (SCA)   The unexpected natural death from a cardiac cause within a short period of time from the onset of symptoms in a person without any prior condition that would appear fatal. See also **sudden cardiac death**.

sudden cardiac death (SCD)   The unexpected natural death from a cardiac cause within a short period of time from the onset of symptoms in a person without any prior condition that would appear fatal. See also **sudden cardiac arrest**.

Sudden Onset   An SVT discrimination algorithm available in certain ICDs which discriminates on the basis of how quickly a tachycardia starts. Using a programmable delta, the ICD compares nontachycardia intervals to the tachycardia intervals to see if the tachycardia started abruptly. If sudden onset is determined, the ICD diagnoses VT. On the other hand, if sudden onset is not found, the ICD diagnoses SVT.

supraventricular   Describes the area above the ventricles of the heart. Typically used to refer to rhythm disorders which originate above the ventricles, that is, in the atria or AV node. Note that while a supraventricular arrhythmia originates above the ventricles, it may affect both atria and ventricles.

supraventricular tachycardia (SVT)   Any type of too-fast heart rhythm which originates above the ventricles, that is, in the atria or AV node. It typically involves an atrial tachycardia which conducts to the ventricles, causing a rapid ventricular response. Supraventricular tachycardia can be automatic (that is, caused by a metabolic disorder, pulmonary disease, or some sort of drug or alcohol toxicity) or reentrant.

sustained   Any arrhythmia that has a duration of 30 seconds or longer. See also **nonsustained**.

SVT   Supraventricular tachycardia.

SVT discrimination   The characteristic of an ICD which allows it to use certain algorithms (SVT discriminators) to help differentiate rapid ventricular rates caused by VT from those caused by an SVT.

SVT discriminator   An algorithm used for SVT discrimination. Examples are **Rate Branch, Sudden Onset, Interval Stability,** and **Morphology Discrimination**.

sweep speed   The speed of an ECG or EGM, usually programmable with a default setting of 25 mm/second.

synchronous   Describes any output pulse (low-voltage or high-voltage) which is timed with respect to some native activity in the patient's heart. Synchronous pacing modes sense intrinsic activity and pace (or inhibit) accordingly.

systole   The period in the cardiac cycle during which one chamber of the heart contracts. The normal heart beat has an atrial systole followed by a ventricular systole. See also **diastole**.

systolic function   The heart's ability to pump blood.

tach   Abbreviation common in ICD programming for tachycardia.

Tach A   An ICD zone programming category which defines slower-rate ventricular tachycardias. Sometimes called 'Slow VT.'

Tach B   An ICD zone programming category which defines faster-rate ventricular tachycardias. Sometimes called 'Fast VT.'

tach zone   A programmed range used by the ICD to detect a ventricular tachycardia. For an ICD, any therapy delivery to a tach zone is called cardioversion.

tachyarrhythmia   Any type of heart rhythm disorder in which the heart beats too quickly. **tachycardia** is a synonym.

tachycardia   Any type of heart rhythm disorder in which the heart beats too quickly. **tachyarrhythmia** is a synonym.

tachy detection rate   A programmable parameter which defines for the ICD the lowest rate which it should consider indicative of a tachyarrhythmia.

tachycardia diagnostics   A broad category of diagnostic data which relate to defibrillation therapy. Examples of tachycardia diagnostics include therapy summary, detect summary, and some electrograms (if they relate to a tachycardia). See also **bradycardia diagnostics**.

tachycardia lead   See **high-voltage lead**. Also called **defibrillation lead**.

tachycardia redetection   The ability of the ICD to determine that an arrhythmia (tachycardia or fibrillation) persists immediately following therapy delivery. The device can be programmed to continue delivering therapy (or deliver more aggressive therapy) if this occurs.

terminate   To end a certain type of heart rhythm. The goal of defibrillation is to terminate ventricular fibrillation. See also **convert**.

therapy delivery   1. A euphemism for the delivery

of a shock or a large amount of energy to the heart by the ICD in order to convert a potentially dangerous ventricular tachyarrhythmia. 2. Any therapeutic response by the ICD to an arrhythmia, including ATP or lower-energy shocks.

therapy summary A form of diagnostic data which shows information on all therapies delivered or aborted.

thoracotomy An open-chest procedure which involves separating the rib cage to expose the heart. Early ICD implantation required a thoracotomy.

tiered therapy The ability of a full-featured ICD to offer different therapeutic responses to different types of arrhythmia, for instance ATP for slow VT, cardioversion for fast VT, and defibrillation for VF.

tilt The percentage drop in voltage from the leading edge (start) of the defibrillation waveform to the trailing edge (end).

titanium A very light metal, much stronger than steel, which is used in ICD and pacemaker cases because of its physical properties and its biocompatibility.

torsades-de-pointes Taken from the French for 'twisting points,' a type of triggered automatic tachycardia which looks like a series of rapid ventricular waves 'turning' on the ECG. Torsades-de-pointes is not caused by an electrical disorder and does not respond to defibrillation.

train In ATP, a pattern of several bursts with or without extrastimuli.

transvenous lead Any lead for an ICD or pacemaker which is passed through a vein and maneuvered into place in the heart.

Trendelenburg position A position for surgical procedures in which the patient lies supine on a table and the table is tilted such that the patient's feet are higher than his or her head. The Trendelenburg position encourages veins around the heart and neck to fill with blood and thus be plumper and more easy to access and dissect.

trigger An event or other criterion which causes the ICD to store an electrogram according to programmed data (that is, single-channel, dual-channel, and so on).

triggered automaticity. An event which precipitates an automatic tachycardia. A typical (but not only) trigger might be a bradycardia pause in the heart rhythm. The trigger accelerates phase 4 of the action potential which, in turn, causes the heart to initiate the next depolarization too quickly after the repolarization. See also **torsades-de-pointes**.

troubleshooting The systematic approach to trying to identify the cause of unexpected and possibly inappropriate ICD behavior with the objective of correcting it.

UBD Use-before date.

UB date Use-before date.

Use-before date (UBD or UB date) A date on the device package before which the device should be implanted. The UB date marks the point at which the housekeeping current drain on the battery may impact stated longevity projections for the device. A device that has passed its UB date may have a shorter service life than a device before or at its UB date.

ventricular electrogram An electrogram from the ICD's ventricular channel only. This is a form of single-channel EGM.

VF Ventricular fibrillation

ventricular fibrillation (VF) A dangerous ventricular arrhythmia characterized by very rapid and wildly disorganized ventricular beats at rates of 200–300 beats a minute. During VF, no individually distinct QRS complexes appear on the ECG.

ventricular paced refractory period A programmable pacemaker parameter which determines an absolute refractory period initiated by a ventricular output pulse.

ventricular tachycardia (VT) A broad term for any too-fast heart rhythms originating in the ventricles, usually at rates between 100 and 300 beats a minute. At high rates, ventricular tachycardia differentiates itself from ventricular fibrillation by the fact that ventricular tachycardia presents identifiable QRS complexes on the ECG, while ventricular fibrillation does not.

voltage The electromotive force as measured in the difference between potentials. ICD output is sometimes measured in volts (V).

VT Ventricular tachycardia.

VVI A pacemaker mode which paces in the ventricle, senses in the ventricle, and inhibits an output in response to sensed activity.

VVIR. A pacemaker mode which paces in the ventricle, senses in the ventricle, inhibits an output in response to sensed activity, and has rate response.

wand   See **programming wand**.

Wolff–Parkinson–White syndrome   A tachycardia caused by a macro-reentry circuit in which the reentry pathway connects the atrium directly to the ventricle.

WPW   Wolff–Parkinson–White syndrome.

zone   See **detection zone**.

Index

Note: page numbers in *italics* refer to figures; those in **bold** to tables.

abdominal implants 17
ablation 123
  conditions responding to 23
  reentry VT 9
  SVTs 7
aborted therapy 52, *53*, 123
  diagnostics 96, *97*, **99**
  vs. missed therapy 116
action potential 2–4, 123
adaptive 123
AF *see* atrial fibrillation
AF Suppression™ algorithm 90, *91*
American College of Cardiology 20
American Heart Association 20
anion 123
annotations 77–8, 123
anti-arrhythmic drugs 115
anticoagulation 26
antitachycardia pacing (ATP) 43, 50,
  55–8, *59*, 123
  atrial, for AF 87
  stored EGM *84*
  tachy redetection after 46, *48*, 58
  terminology **57**
  Therapy Summary 94–6
  troubleshooting 117
arrhythmias 123
  detection *see* detection
  EGM storage 81
  induction, DFT testing 31
  redetection 46, *48*
  sudden cardiac death 1
  therapy 50–61
asynchronous 123
asystole 123
AT/AF Burden Trends 89
ATP *see* antitachycardia pacing
atrial fibrillation (AF) 7, 62, 123
  discrimination 63–4
  management 87–90
  paroxysmal 7, 130
  permanent 7, 131
  persistent 7, 131

troubleshooting 119
atrial flutter 123
  discrimination 63
  troubleshooting 119
atrial tachycardia (AT) 62, 63, 65, 123
atrial tracking 72
attempt **57**, 123
autodecrementing *see* ramping, ATP
Autointrinsic Conduction Search
  (AICS) 87, *90*
automatic implantable cardioverter-
  defibrillator (AICD) 12
automatic implantable defibrillator
  (AID) 12
automaticity 4–5, 124
  triggered 4–5, 135
auto(matic) mode switch (AMS) 72,
  74, 87–9, 100–102, **103**
Auto Sensitivity algorithm 37–9, *40*
Auto Update Morphology Template
  110
AV delay 71, **73**, 124
AV nodal reentrant tachycardia
  (AVNRT) 6–7, 124

base rate, pacemaker 70–71, **73**, 124
batteries 16–17
  low, indicators 104, 107
  voltage checks 108
beats per minute (bpm) 124
bin 45, 124
binning 45–6, *48*, 124
biphasic waveform 33, 52–4, 124
bleeding off 52, 124
bradyarrhythmia 124
bradycardia 124
  diagnostics 100–103, 124
  parameters, programming 27, 34,
  70–76
Brugada syndrome 9, 23, 24, 124
burst 56, 57, 124
burst cycle length (BCL) 56–7, 124
bypass tract 5–6, 124

can 18, 124
capacitance 50, 124–5

capacitor 17, 50, 125
  maintenance 50–51, 125
  reformation 50–51
capture 109, 125
  tests 28, *29*, 109–10, *111*, 117, 125
  threshold *29*, 109, 125
cardiac arrest survivors 21, 22, 24
Cardiac Compass 89
cardiac resynchronization therapy
  (CRT) 125
  with defibrillation (CRT-D) 70, 126
  in pacemaker system (CRT-P) 126
cardiac transplantation
  heart failure patients not eligible for
  23–4
  patients awaiting 22
cardiomyopathy 1, 125
cardioversion 17, 43, 50, 58, 125
case, ICD 18
cation 125
Centers for Medicare and Medicaid
  Services (CMS) 20, 125
cephalic cutdown 28, 125
charge times 27, 31, 52, *53*, 125
chest X-ray 34, 104, 117
clipping, stored EGMs 81
coils 18, 34, 125
committed ICDs 52, 125
components, ICD 16–19
connector 126
convert 126
coronary artery bypass grafting
  (CABG) 23
coronary artery disease (CAD)
  ICD indications 21, 22, 23
  sudden cardiac death 1

DDD pacing 70, 72, 126
DDDR pacing 70, 126
Decay Delay 39, *40*
default value 126
defib 126
Defib Off 46–7, 126
Defib Only 43–4, **45**, 126
defibrillation 16, 43, 50, 126
defibrillation lead *see* high-voltage lead

defibrillation threshold (DFT) 51–2,
    126
  energy output for therapy and 51–2
  high 32–4, 128
  testing 27, 31–2, 51, 127
defibrillator status line 78, 126
Defib with single tach zone 44, 126
Defib with Tach A or Tach B 44–7,
    126
DEFINITE trial 20
deformation 50, 126
depolarization 2–3, 126
detection (arrhythmia) 43–9, 126
  bins 45, 126–7
  data 93–4
  vs. sensing 41
  zones 43, 44, 127
Detection Summary 93–4, 99, 127
device, ICD 16–19
  preparation for implantation 27–8
  replacement 104, 107
device-based testing (DBT) 29–34,
    117, 127
device configuration 43, 127
DFT see defibrillation threshold
diagnosis 81, 127
Diagnosis Information 94, 95, 127
diagnostics (including diagnostic data)
    93–105, 127
  bradycardia 100–103, 124
  episode 96–7, 98, 127
  erasure 93
  lifetime 97, 99, 99, 129
  shortcuts 104
  tachycardia 93–7, 99, 134
  troubleshooting 116, 118
diastole 127
diastolic function 127
documentation
  diagnostic data 93, 104
  follow-up 111, 112
  at implantation 34
double-counting 118–19, 127
downsizing, ICD 14
driving 113
drug therapy 115
dual-chamber ICDs 17, 18–19, 127
  implantation 28
  pacing diagnostics 100–102
  sensing 39–41
  SVT discrimination 63, 64
dual-channel electrograms 80, 127
Dump Capacitors 52
dynamic range 81, 127

ECG filter 79, 127
education, patient 112–13
EGMs see electrograms

ejection fraction, left ventricular
    see left ventricular ejection
    fraction
elective replacement indicator 107,
    127
electrical heterogeneity 2, 127
electrocardiogram (ECG) 77, 78, 79
electrograms (EGM) 77–85, 127
  arrhythmia detection 43, 45–6, 47,
    48
  atrial 77, 80, 123
  capture test 110, 111
  dual-channel 80, 127
  near- and far-field 80, 81
  real-time 77–9, 108, 132
  stored 77, 79–82, 83, 84, 133
    diagnostics 93, 104
    troubleshooting 116, 118
  ventricular 77, 80, 135
electrophysiological (EP) study 21,
    22, 117
energy
  cardioversion 50
  defibrillation 16, 50
  delivered 52, 126
  programming, for therapy 51–2
  stored 52, 133
epicardial leads 13, 14, 17, 127
  pediatric patients 18
episode(s) 93, 127
  Detection Summary 93–4
  Diagnosis Information 94, 95
  diagnostics 96–7, 98, 127
Event Histogram 100, 101, 103, 127–8
extrastimulus 57, 128

familial disorders 22
fib zone 43–4, 128
fixed 128
fixed pulse width 54–5, 128
fixed tilt 54–5, 128
fluoroscopy 128
follow-up 106–14
  automated 106, 123–4
  Auto Update Morphology Template
    110
  capture testing 109–10
  documentation 111
  high-voltage lead integrity check
    110–111
  interrogation 106–8
  patients' questions 112–13
  programming 111–12
  real-time EGM 108
  real-time measurements 108

gain 77, 128
Guidant devices 33

guidelines 20, 128

header 16, 18, 128
heart failure 23–4, 128
Heart Rate Histogram 100, 101, 128
Heart Rhythm Society 20
Heilman, Stephen 12
High Voltage Charging 96
high-voltage lead (defibrillation lead)
    17–19, 126, 128
  impedance 30, 111
  insertion 28
  integrity check (HVLIC) 30, 110–
    111, 117
  testing 117
high-voltage (high-energy) therapy
    50–55
  inappropriate 62, 117–19, 120
  patient's questions 113
  special features 86–7, 88, 89
history of ICDs 12–15
housekeeping current 27, 128
hypertrophic cardiomyopathy 22
hysteresis 71, 73, 128
  with search 71, 73

identification bracelets 113
impedance, lead 117
  changes 104, 108
  defibrillation lead 30, 111
  pacing lead 29, 108
implantable atrial cardioverter-
    defibrillators 7
implantation site 26
implant procedure 26–36
  conclusion 34
  defibrillation threshold testing
    31–2
  device-based testing 29–31
  high defibrillation threshold 32–4
  history 13, 17, 26
  lead testing 28–9
  postoperative care 34
  preparation for 26–7
  prior to 26
  team 27–8
  venous access 28
inappropriate therapy 62, 117–19,
    120, 128
incidence 128
indications 20–25
  Class I 21–2, 125
  Class IIa 22, 125
  Class IIb 22–3, 125
  Class III 125, –2423
  class system 20
inherited disorders 22
inter 128

interference, device 115–16, 118
interrogation 106–8, 128
interval 44, 129
  average *48*, 124
  averaging 44, *45*
  counting 44–5
  current *48*, 126
  pre-trigger 81, 131
Interval Stability 63–4, 129
intra 129
intracardiac electrograms (IEGM)
      77, 129
  see also electrograms
ion 129

joules (J) 51, 129

leads 17–19
  extraction 107
  impedance *see* impedance, lead
  insertion 28
  problems 107, 117
  replacement 107
  testing 28–9, 117
  see also epicardial leads; high-
      voltage lead; pacing leads
left ventricular dysfunction 21, 22
left ventricular ejection fraction
      (LVEF) 129
  indication for ICD 22
  sudden cardiac death and 1
lifetime diagnostics 97, **99**, *99*, 129
lithium 16, 129
lithium-iodide cell 16, 129
lithium-vanadium cell 16, 129
long QT syndrome (LQTS) 8, 22, 24,
      129
Lown, Bernard 12

macro-reentry 7, 129
MADIT trial 20
MADIT II trial 20
magnets 115–16, 118
manual 129
manufacturer's representative 27, 129
mapping 129
maximum duration 82, 129
maximum time to diagnosis (MTD)
      46, 66–8, 87, *89*
maximum time to fib (MTF) 46,
      66–8, 86–7, *88*
maximum tracking rate (MTR) 72,
      73, 129
Medtronic devices 33
membrane potential 2, 129
micro-reentry 6–7, 130
microwave oven 113
Mirowski, Mieczyslaw (Michel) 12–14

Mirowski Award 13
Mirowski Symposium 13
mode, pacing 70–74, **73**, 130
mode switching 72, 87–9, 100–102,
      103
mode switch log 102, **103**, 130
monitoring, remote systems 19, 90–91
monophasic waveform 33, 52–4, 130
morphology 130
Morphology Discrimination 65–6, *67*,
      110, 119, 130
Mower, Morton 12
myocardial infarction (MI) 130
  prior, ICD indications 21, 22
  reentrant VT/VF after 9
myocardium 130

navigation 130
New York Heart Association (NYHA)
      classification 130
nominal value 130
noncommitted ICDs 52, *53*, 96, 130
noninvasive programmed stimulation
      (NIPS) 117
nonsustained 130
normal sinus rhythm (NST) 130
  detection 43, 44
North American Society of Pacing and
      Electrophysiology (NASPE)
      (now Heart Rhythm Society)
      20

oversensing 37, 43

pacemaker-mediated tachycardia
      (PMT) 72–3
  detection rate 73, **74**
  options 72–3, **74**
pacemakers 16
pacing 17, 70–76
  asynchronous 70
  atrial overdrive 89–90, *91*
  competitive 70, 125
  diagnostic data 100–103
  dual-chamber 72
  episodal 74–5, 127
  initial 34
  mode and timing parameters
      70–74
  post-shock (PSP) 75–6, 131
  special features 87, *90*
  states 100, 130
  temporary 108
  see also bradycardia
pacing leads 18–19
  impedance *29*, 108
  testing 117
pacing system analyzer (PSA) 27, 130

parameter settings
  at implantation 27
  programming *see* programming
  verifying 117
patch leads *see* epicardial leads
Patient Alert 90
patients
  questions, answering 112–13
  special ICD features 90–91
pediatric patients 18
pharmacological therapy 115
physical activities 112–13
physicians, other 113
PMT *see* pacemaker-mediated
      tachycardia
polarity
  programmable 131
  reversing 34, 55
port 131
port plug 19, 131
postoperative care 34
post-shock pacing (PSP) 75–6, 131
post-ventricular atrial refractory
      period (PVARP) 72, **73**
premature ventricular contractions
      (PVC) 44, 72, 100, 131
premature ventricular events (PVE)
      100, 131
pre-trigger interval 81, 131
prevalence 131
primary prevention 131
  trials 20–21, 131
programmer 19, 131
programming
  diagnostic data erasure 93
  at follow-up 111–12
  initial 27–8, 34
  temporary 108
  wand 27, 30, 106–7, 131
psychiatric illness 23
pulses per minute (ppm) 70–71, 131
PVC *see* premature ventricular
      contractions
PVC options 72, **74**
PV delay 71–2, **73,** 131
P-wave, lead testing 28, *29*

QRS morphology 65–6, 110
questions, patients' 112–13

ramp 131–2
ramping, ATP 57–8, *59*
ramp step *58*, 132
Rate Branch 63, *64*, 132
rate-responsive AV delay (RRAVD)
      132
rate-responsive AV/PV delay 72, **73**
rate-responsive ICDs 71, 132

rate-responsive ventricular refractory
    period **74**
Rate Smoothing 87
readaptation **57,** 132
real-time measurements 108, *109,* 132
record-keeping *see* documentation
redetection 46, *48,* 132
    ATP therapy 58
    sinus 81–2, 133
reentrant 132
reentry 2, 5–6, 132
reformation 50–51, 132
refractory 3, 132
refractory period
    absolute 72, 123
    post-pace 41
    post-ventricular atrial (PVARP) 72,
        73
    rate-responsive ventricular **74**
    relative 72, 132
    sensed 38
    shortest **74**
    ventricular paced 72, **73,** 135
remote monitoring systems 19, 90–91
replacement, device 104, 107
repolarization 3, 132
representative, manufacturer's 27, 129
rescue 50, 132
rest rate 71, **73,** 132
right bundle branch block,
        unexplained SCD with 23
risk factors 132–3
R-on-T phenomenon 70, 131
R-wave
    automatic sensitivity algorithms 38,
        39
    lead testing 28, *29*

safety margin 133
scanning, ATP 57–8, *59,* 133
SCD-HeFT trial 20–21
sedation 27, 31
self-terminate 133
self-terminated arrhythmias 52, *53*
sensing 37–42, 133
    problems 116, 118–19
    see also oversensing; undersensing
sensitivity 37, 133
    adjustments 117, 119
    automatic algorithms 37–9, 40–41
    maximum 39–40
sensor **74,** 133
sensor histogram 102–3, 133
sexual activity 113
shocking vectors 34, 55, 133
    programmable 131
shocks 113, 133
    see also high-voltage therapy

sick sinus syndrome 99
single-chamber ICDs 17, 133
    implantation 28
    pacing states 100
    SVT discrimination 64
sinoatrial (SA) node 4
sinus redetection 81–2, 133
sinus rhythm 133
    normal *see* normal sinus rhythm
sinus tachycardia 63, 65
size, ICD *14,* 17
sodium ions 2
sodium-potassium pump 4
special events 82, 133
special features 86–92
specificity 133
sports 112
St Jude Medical devices 33–4
    AF Suppression™ algorithm 90, *91*
    detection **44,** 45, 46
    real-time EGMs 78
    sensing 37–40
ST-segment elevations, unexplained
        SCD with 22–3
subclavian stick 28, 133
substrate 9, 133
sudden cardiac arrest (SCA) *see*
        sudden cardiac death
sudden cardiac death (SCD) 1–11,
        134
    family history 22–3
    survivors 21, 22
Sudden Onset 65, 134
support groups, patient 113
supraventricular 134
supraventricular tachycardia (SVT)
        6, 134
    discrimination 62–9, 118, 119, 134
    discriminators 62–9, 117, 134
    maximum time to diagnosis (MTD)
        87
    with rapid ventricular response 7
sustained 134
SVT *see* supraventricular tachycardia
sweep speed 79, 134
swimming 113
synchronous 134
syncope 24
    in advanced structural heart disease
        23
    troubleshooting **120**
    unexplained 21, 22–3, 23
system, ICD 16–19
    see also device, ICD
systole 134
systolic function 22, 134

tach 134

Tach A 44, 134
Tach B 44, 134
tachyarrhythmia 134
tachycardia 134
    automatic 4, 124
    diagnostics 93–7, **99,** 134
    episodes 74
    lead *see* high-voltage lead
    pacemaker-mediated *see*
        pacemaker-mediated
        tachycardia
    parameters, programming 27,
        30–31
    redetection 134
    reentry 5–6
    sinus 63, 65
    types 6–10
    see also specific types
tachy detection rates 44, 72, 134
    troubleshooting 117, 118, 119
tach zones 44–5, 134
team, implantation 27–8
telemetry 19, 30, 107
terminal illness 23
terminate 134
therapy 50–61
    aborted *see* aborted therapy
    delivery 50, 52, 62, 134–5
    EGM storage 81
    failure to deliver 115–17, **120**
    high-voltage *see* high-voltage
        therapy
    inappropriate 62, 117–19, **120,** 128
    tiered 43, 135
    verifying settings 117
Therapy Summary 94–6, **99,** 135
thoracotomy (open-chest surgery) 13,
        17, 26, 135
Threshold Start 38, 39–40
tiered therapy 43, 135
tilt 33–4, 54–5, 135
    fixed 54–5, 128
titanium 18, 135
torsades-de-pointes 5, 8–9, 135
train 56, 57, 135
training 86
transtelephonic monitoring (TTM)
        90–91
transvenous leads 17–19, 135
    see also leads
travel 113
Trendelenburg position 26, 135
trigger 81, 135
troubleshooting 115–21, 135
    failure to deliver therapy 115–17
    inappropriate therapy delivery
        117–19
    matrix **120**

2:1 blocking rate **73**

undersensing 37, 43, 116
Update Trends 108, *109*
use-before-date (UBD or UB date)
 27, 135

venous access, ICD implantation 28
ventricular fibrillation (VF) 7–8, 135
 detection 43–6
 incessant 23
 induced 21
 redetection 46
 reentry 9–10
 survivors 21, 22
 SVT discrimination 62–9
 therapy 50–55
ventricular tachycardia (VT) 135

cardiac arrest survivors 21
detection 43, 44–7, *48*
failure to deliver therapy
 115, 116
hemodynamically stable 128
ICD indications 21, 22, 23
incessant 23
monomorphic 7, *8*, 130
nonsustained (NSVT) 7, 130
 ICD indications 21, 22
polymorphic 7, *8*, 131
redetection 46, *48*
reentry 9–10, 55–6
slow 44, 58, 63, 100, 118
sustained 7
 inducible 21, 22
 spontaneous 21, 22
SVT discrimination 62–9

therapy 50–58
Ventritex device 33–4
VF *see* ventricular fibrillation
voltage 51, 135
voltage multipliers 16
VT *see* ventricular tachycardia
VVI pacing 70, 72, 135
VVIR pacing 70, 135

wand, programming 27, 30, 106–7,
 131
warning indicators 90, 104, 107
Watkins, Levi 13
waveform morphologies 52–5
Wolff–Parkinson–White (WPW)
 syndrome 7, 135–6

zones, detection 43, 44, 127

Printed and bound by CPI Group (UK) Ltd, Croydon, CR0 4YY

27/10/2024

14580395-0005

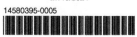